D0120959

NG

BACK

TROUBLE

Consumers' Association
publishers of **Which?**
14 Buckingham Street
London WC2N 6DS

a Consumer Publication

edited by Edith Rudinger

published by Consumers' Association
publishers of **Which?**

Consumer Publications are
available from Consumers'
Association and from
booksellers. Titles of other
Consumer Publications are
given at the end of this book.

© Consumers' Association October 1975
reprinted January 1976

ISBN 0 85202 103 8

-2 FEB 1994

 Computer typeset
and printed offset litho
by Page Bros (Norwich) Ltd

CONTENTS

Foreword

Background *page* 1

This book tells you about the spine and what can go wrong with it, concentrating mainly on the lower back—the lumbar region of the spine. It also advises on ways of avoiding back trouble and, for those who suffer from backache or sciatic pain already, offers some guidance on how to ease it, if not actually get rid of it. The facts are as accurate as present knowledge allows. But the deductions and the practical applications will change as new facts emerge and back pain research gets into its stride. If more were known about back pain and what can cause it, it would not be such a problem; we should be better at preventing it and you might not be reading this book.

BACKGROUND

In the majority of cases, back pain arises from some minor mechanical derangement of the spine, not a serious disease in itself, however bad the pain may be in an acute attack. In other words, it will not kill or endanger life even if it is cripplingly painful. But you should get your doctor's advice if the pain is severe, or lasts more than three to four days: back pain may be due to disease of some other part of the body, and the doctor must find out whether this is so in your case.

For most people, the occasional backache is quite normal. Just as muscles become painful and tender after the first game of the season, or your arms would ache after hand-milking a cow for the first time, so does the back after work for which it is out of training.

Back pain is related to the effort involved in a particular activity. This is not necessarily a matter of how heavy the work is so much as the awkwardness of the job and how often it has to be repeated. For example, it is easier and needs less effort to lift and carry small heavy loads with good handles than a large bulky load of a quarter the weight with nowhere to grasp it. Lifting infrequently can cause as much back trouble as lifting too much if it is done so seldom that you are never in training for it. The young may get away with it by virtue of being generally fit, but as one gets older and the spine is subjected to wear and tear, the regularity with which manual work is done becomes more important. Someone engaged in heavy manual work who lacks skill is at risk from the cumulative effects of frequent minor injury, while a really skilful person may safely handle equally heavy loads without fear of injury. At work and at home, training is worthwhile in order to reduce the amount of stress that, often quite unnecessarily, is put on the spine. Become more skilful and the same job can be done with less effort and less risk.

Not that handling loads is the only cause of back pain. Postural stress arising from muscular fatigue is another cause; it is at least as common, and it is avoidable. Millions of people get backache every day, leaning over machinery, working at sinks or when sitting still. By re-designing the working environment, much of the postural stress which leads to backache could be eliminated.

One of the many things about back pain which is puzzling is why it should have become so much commoner. It has been said that man has not yet adapted to an erect stance and that the spine is not designed for it, and it is suggested that the evolutionary transition from being a quadruped is incomplete and inefficient. But man and his immediate ancestors appear to have been upright for millions of years, which should have been long enough.

Back pain seems to be a feature of technically advanced communities in which people have also become less tolerant of pain. Moreover, life has become comparatively more complex and it is perhaps not surprising that backache, like headache, can become worse as a result of psychological stress, such as anxiety, bereavement and other social and emotional pressures.

Little is known of why one man should be the victim of back trouble while another is not, although there are a number of minor anomalies in the spine which are associated with a marginally greater likelihood of trouble. Tallness rather than shortness is also linked to a marginally increased susceptibility to back trouble—but there is no cure for that. In some cases, the tendency to back trouble seems to run in families and some developmental weaknesses in the spine are of genetic origin. There are some races in whom certain spinal disorders are common. But it is not easy to say whether those people who have vulnerable backs have acquired them genetically or simply because they do things in the same way physically as their forefathers.

Back pain has been starved of scientific attention. Diagnosing the actual cause of back pain today is rather like the diagnosis of anaemia before the development of all the laboratory tests which are now taken for granted. What is known about back pain stems from doctors' experience of what patients tell them about it and from what they find on examination. It also comes from the observations which the surgeon makes during an operation, and their relationship to the previous symptoms and examination pre-operatively, and the relief of pain afterwards. The acumen, skill and understanding of individual doctors and surgeons can be great, but their knowledge is mainly empirical. Back pain is a distressingly common problem, and one which will not be solved by tomorrow lunchtime. The main task is to tackle prevention.

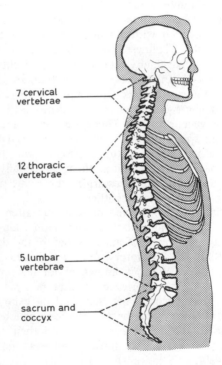

7 cervical vertebrae

12 thoracic vertebrae

5 lumbar vertebrae

sacrum and coccyx

The spine consists of bones and ligaments, muscles and tendons. It contains the spinal cord and the nerve roots which emerge from it. Each of the bones of the spine is called a vertebra. Between the bodies of the vertebrae is the intervertebral disc, a thick piece of tissue of great strength which can change shape as the vertebral bodies on either side of it move.

The spine is very mobile: it can bend forwards, backwards and sideways, and it can rotate. The cervical (neck) and lumbar regions are the most mobile, the thoracic (chest) region being restricted by the rib cage. Forward and backward movements are free in both the lumbar and cervical spine, and to a less extent, so is sideways motion. Rotation is greatest in the cervical region, less in the thoracic, again because of the rib cage, and least in the lumbar region.

Almost all the spinal movements are related to movement of other parts of the body. Movement of the head in relation to the chest brings about movement in the cervical spine and in the upper thoracic region. Movement of the thoracic spine is produced mainly as a result of actions of the upper limbs in relation to the trunk. Lumbar movement is determined by movements of the upper part of the trunk in relation to the pelvis and therefore indirectly by actions of the upper limbs relative to the lower limbs. There is obviously more to it than that: witness the lumbar mobility due to pelvic movements of a belly-dancer. Generally, however, it is the relationship between the trunk and the lower limbs that matters. Even straightening the knees when sitting moves the lumbar spine.

In fact, the spine is never still. It moves with every breath because of expansion of the rib cage: breathe in deeply and the thoracic spine straightens; exhale fully and it flexes forwards.

The spine can take very great stresses. They arise from the direct effect of the force of gravity on the body and the muscular activity needed to resist the force of gravity and to produce or stop movement, and from forces applied from outside the body.

The earth's gravitational field imposes a constant force on us. Lying down, the vertical force on the spine is obviously minimal. Standing erect, very little muscular activity is needed in order to keep in equilibrium. The load on the spine is almost solely due to the effect of gravity on the head and arms and the upper part of the trunk, and is taken mainly by the vertebral bodies and discs.

muscular activity

The force of gravity and muscular activity are the main sources of the energy which produces spinal movement. Bend down, and you rely on gravity to do part of the work, using muscles to control and stop the descent. Straighten up, and muscles must do all the work, and against gravity.

The function of a muscle is to develop tension between two bony points and prevent their being pulled apart, or to control the rate at which they are being pulled apart, or, by shortening, to draw them together. Without muscular support, the spine is inherently unstable—as in an unconscious person. The muscles which support the spine are those of the back and neck, together with the muscles of the trunk.

Of the muscles attached directly to the spine, the short deep ones close to the vertebrae control the movements and posture between adjacent vertebrae. The more superficial back muscles, the ones you can feel, are longer and control a larger region; they are active in straightening the spine and arching it back and in holding the posture when leaning forwards.

The abdominal muscles help your spine to bend by pulling the front of the rib cage closer to the pelvis. Abdominal muscles also control twisting actions between the shoulders and the pelvis—no golfer could do without them—and they are used when pushing and for holding the posture when leaning backwards. When you bend sideways, they share the work with the back muscles on that side. Good abdominal muscles are important in the prevention of backache.

There is another mechanism by which the muscles of the trunk support the spine, indirectly. This is by the involuntary increase in pressure inside the chest and within the abdomen. Increased pressure in the abdomen helps to prevent the front of the rib cage approaching the pelvis, and so either stops further forward bending or helps the back muscles to straighten up.

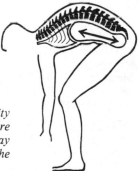

the arrow in the abdominal cavity shows how an increase in pressure helps to push the rib cage away from the pelvis and so support the spine during lifting

There is also a muscle called psoas (from the greek word for loin), originating from the sides and front of the lumbar vertebral bodies, which flexes the hip joints. When active, it pulls on the spine, compressing the discs; when you are sitting still, it gives the spine postural support.

If you start to lean forwards, the muscles of the back become active and tense in order to counter the effects of gravity on the upper half of the body which is now forward of the hips, so that the trunk is canti-levered from the pelvis. To keep leaning forwards, the spine is held by the pull of the back muscles between the vertebrae and the pelvis and this pull is countered

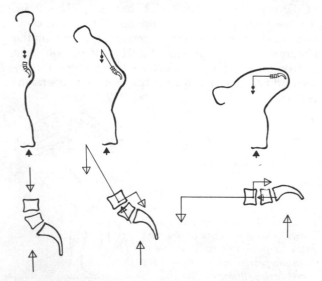

the effects of gravity on stress at the lumbar spine in differ-ent postures

by a force which compresses the vertebral bodies and discs. The muscles of the hip, thigh and back are strongly active to hold the trunk in the horizontal position. As you come upright again, the muscle tension and resulting compressive force increase in order to produce the necessary movement.

Any muscular activity and movement is likely to cause an increase in spinal stress. Stand on some bathroom scales; then, watching the pointer, raise your arms and you will see it move up as your arms lift. The force needed to lift the arms is reflected down your spine to your feet and via the scales to the floor. And similarly with every other activity— pushing, pulling, carrying, getting up, sitting down, and anything else you can think of. For example, to drive a golf ball, the golfer has to twist his whole trunk, and the work of swinging trunk, arms and club and hitting the ball is reflected by an equal and opposite twisting force (axial torque) in the spine. If you do not believe that this torque is transmitted all the way down the spine via the pelvis to the feet, just try the same movement when standing on a revolving platform or on a sheet of ice.

Stress on the spine also arises when body movements are caused by outside forces. Riding a bicycle or a horse, sitting on a tractor, or jolting about in cars, lorries or motorbuses, every movement imparted to you is resisted. Taking a tractor over a ploughed field, every rut and every stone over which one wheel of the tractor rides will produce a vertical acceleration and, because it is one-sided, a sideways jolt. Even the lateral force of a car turning a corner at speed offers a sideways force to be resisted—and most car seats give poor lateral support.

Falls, jars, jolts, and stumblings are common and would cause more injury to the spine were it not for the spine's function of shock absorption. It works in two ways: dissipating the energy by converting it into movement and altering the quality of the applied force so that it is less likely to cause injury.

The function of converting force into movement is a vital one. Unless some of the applied energy can be quickly converted into movement, it will break bones or cause other injury. In young and supple people, much more movement can be produced than in someone old and stiff, and they can therefore take more punishment than the elderly. As well as being more mobile, the vertebrae in the young spine can bend or change shape more readily in response to loads and muscular tension. This is why the young are better than old people at taking the jerk (the rate of increase in force) and reducing it.

Just by looking at someone, you cannot say how much work and of what kind he will be fit for. Heavy people, by virtue of larger muscles and bones, should be stronger than small ones. Those who are hugely fat have more weight to throw about, and can shift things easily by simply leaning on them, though they may get a bit short of breath. Otherwise, there is not much to go on. If a person is normally active and free from disease, he should be physically capable of any reasonable task, given the right training and the acquisition of the proper skill. Muscular training, coordination and skill matter more than anything else, and together can overcome minor weaknesses or stiffening in the spine itself.

Spinal functions also include a safety mechanism: namely, protective backache or pain. This is mainly of value in giving warning of postural stress. It is not so good at preventing injury due to straining the back when something proves too heavy or unexpectedly will not move because it is stuck—then the pain may come too late. Generally, the spine is like any other part of the body when put to work for which it is unfit: it warns you not to overdo it.

Avoiding spinal stress
Although the spine is capable of moving in many different directions and of adopting different positions, in some of these positions it is more vulnerable to stress, especially if the position is held for any length of time or the back is required to do a lot of work in such a position. Episodes of back pain of physical origin are related either to postural stress or to the effort involved in handling a load.

The things to avoid are, first, remaining in positions which are likely to cause muscular fatigue and postural stress; and secondly, struggling with anything which cannot be moved readily and quickly, particularly if this involves sideways twisting or one-handed efforts.

Comparatively few people escape getting a bit of back trouble once in a while. If you have had trouble with your back before and know what caused it, you have an idea of how to avoid it happening again. In most cases, the remedy lies in minimising the brief but significant stress on the spine arising from a given piece of work or the prolonged but lesser stress arising from a given posture. Work, in this context, encompasses domestic and recreational activities as well as the work for which one is paid.

Many of the things we use at home and at work—equipment, furniture, storage spaces—are badly designed. There is also room for improvement in the design of working procedures. Ergonomics—the scientific application of the analysis of working situations and design in relation to man's structure, function and behaviour—has a great deal to offer in the prevention of back pain. But while waiting for ergonomists, planners, architects and designers to find the answers to the problem, there are a number of ways we can deal with the situation ourselves.

The first rule in the analysis of any working situation is to define what the job is for and to understand why it has to be done. Part of the ergonomic solution to cleaning dirty floors is to stop them from getting dirty in the first place. Unlike Japan, for instance, in this country it is socially acceptable to wear outdoor shoes in the house and so the dirt of the road gets trampled into the floor coverings.

The ergonomic questions to be answered cover a wide range, such as the instructions given with the job, the mental work involved, the accuracy needed. When one is concerned about spinal stress and backache or back injury, the questions should include

—what are the objectives of the job? why has the job to be done at all, and is there an alternative?

—what, in physical terms, does the job demand? what is the posture? what movements, force and rate of working are needed?

—what are the functional effects on the muscles, heart and lungs? and what mechanical stresses are induced?

—are there any limitations on who is fit for the job, in terms of age, sex, weight and height, strength and mobility?

—what training is needed to achieve the necessary skill, coordination and physical fitness?

posture

'Good' posture is any posture which allows efficient use of the body for a given purpose and is both comfortable (no aches, pains or other symptoms) for as long as the posture is maintained and has no deleterious after-effects. In other words, posture should be efficient in terms of function and not cause mechanical stress. For instance, holding a book at arm's length demands muscle tension in the whole arm to counter the effect of gravity on the arm and the book; holding it at the side of the body needs only finger tension. Leaning forwards over a bench imposes a stress on the spine and muscles of the back and hip of up to four or five times the force of gravity on the upper half of the body. Specialists can calculate postural stress in a given part of the body from the size and shape of the parts of the body and the position in which they are held. From this they can calculate roughly how much muscle tension is needed. They can also compare the work required of the heart and lungs and breathing capacity in different postures. For example, breathing capacity is much less when stooping down with the spine flexed than when upright. Similarly, when the shoulder muscles are used for pushing or holding something up high, the resulting muscle tension has the effect of splinting the rib cage and limiting its movement.

Posture also affects muscle function. A joint at the extreme of one of the ranges of its movement is not in the best position for the muscles to act most efficiently. For instance, the skill and strength of the hands is reduced in extreme positions of the neck.

Good posture can more easily be defined negatively: it should neither cause symptoms for the time it is maintained nor cause any subsequently; it should not prevent the joints of the limbs being in the optimal position for any given task; and it should require no more than a minimal level of muscular activity to maintain it. Good posture can be spoiled by emotional tension, anxiety, anger or fatigue, which cause posturally unnecessary muscle tension.

standing
When standing, the spinal column has a series of curves giving it a sigmoid shape. The natural curvature can vary from person to person. It is when the curves are increased or decreased too much under strain that trouble is more likely to occur.

For a correct stance, lift the top of your head without sticking your chin out—growing tall. As well as standing tall, you have to stand relaxed. Standing still for a long period can be uncomfortable for someone not used to it, and when tired by standing, one tends to increase the fatiguing effect by increasing the tension of the muscles. However, except for soldiers on parade, standing still is rarely necessary. Mostly, we are free to look about, move our hands and shift from one foot to another, and so any given postural stance is seldom maintained for long.

Backache when standing may be due simply to bad design of the work place. One remedy for postural stress is to change position. If you cannot, and the job demands work with one hand, use the other hand to lean on. When you use both hands and are standing at a work bench, table or a sink, ideally you should be able to rest your pelvis or stomach against it with one foot forward in line with your hands, so that you have a balanced posture. If you have to stand back from, say, the sink edge, while working, the angle of the trunk is increased, and so is the stress. Many people with back trouble find that a small footstool to rest one leg on is a help when standing at work.

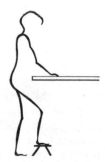

sitting

Sitting still is a more frequent fate than standing still, and there is less room for movement. Backache when sitting is very common, particularly in car drivers, aircraft passengers, theatregoers and tv addicts.

The design of the seat and back rest of a chair should relate to the fundamental question of what the chair is for. Seats for a cinema or theatre or for watching television need to be satisfactory for the visual field of stage or screen and for comfort. Seats in aircraft should be comfortable for reading and eating and looking about, and also help to safeguard passengers in the event of an accident. The seating in inter-city trains is designed to take into account the need for space, so that passengers' sitting postures can be changed. The type of chair designed for typists can be good but, in effect, it is so only in relation to the position of the typewriter and desk or table.

For some other activities, a specially designed chair should be provided. For example, the forward sitting position of a 'cellist or harpist needs a chair designed to support the lower back because perching on an ordinary chair increases backache. For aircraft pilots, the solution was to take the impression of individual spines and make individual back rests. It was found that this relieved pilots with backache of their symptoms and those who had no symptoms pronounced themselves more comfortable.

When sitting for leisure rather than work, some people with back trouble find a high-backed hard chair preferable. The important thing is to get one's bottom well back into the chair because sitting

*poor: low lounging chair with
no lumbar support*

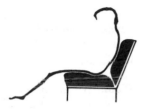

slouched in a chair may flex the lumbar region more than any other movement or posture. Some back sufferers are more comfortable if they avoid crossing their knees and sit with their feet and knees well apart.

If the chair is soft and does not give enough support, put a cushion at the small of the back. Lumbar support is more important than support at shoulder level. If you often use the same chair, it is quite a good idea to put tape or elastic on to both sides of the cushion and fix it to the chair, so that it is there when needed. Choose a chair that is the right height for you and remember that you need room to shift your posture a little within the chair itself, and in the space around it.

—when working
The seat of a chair for working in should be deep enough front to back so that the thighs are supported, and the front edge of the seat should not dig into the thigh (this could cause pressure on the sciatic nerve). The chair seat should be inclined about 5 degrees to the horizontal, backwards, and be high enough for the knee angle to be not less than 90 degrees. It should not slope down into the middle from the sides. This

causes the thigh bones to take weight instead of the pelvic bones which are built for the job.

The back rest should be adjustable so that the height above the seat can be varied to provide support at the lumbar part of the spine. A full-length back rest should be contoured at the lumbar level.

The cushioning and padding should feel firm. As well as taking the sitter's weight, the seat should resist other forces such as those exerted by the sitter when pulling levers and pressing on pedals. In a car, for example, the driver's seat should resist the pressure between the pelvic bones and the back rest when he treads on the brake.

The perfect shape of chair is no good unless it is the right size so that the person's feet are not dangling in mid-air because the chair is too high, nor his knees at chest level because it is too low. The important point is that any seat used for working in should fit the individual using it.

The chairs designed and sold to industrial and commercial organisations are on the whole an improvement on those for living rooms, restaurants, theatres and cinemas, but ergonomically they are only satisfactory if the working environment in which they are used is also well designed. Even with a well-designed working chair which allows one to sit supported in the right places, with the spine in a balanced neutral position and freedom to make regular minor changes in posture, the work itself may make it less than satisfactory.

Just how good a posture is depends chiefly on the purpose for which the posture was adopted. For a

given situation, at work or at leisure, key factors are
  —the angle of vision, and the need for subsidiary
    movements of the head
  —the position of the hands in relation to vision
    and the rest of the body
  —the support of the body.
So as well as sitting or standing properly when
working what matters is what you are doing with
your hands and the forces they are exerting, where
your head has to be to see what needs to be seen, and
what parts of your body are supported.

When work is laid out on a flat surface, the angle
of vision is downwards and it is necessary to bend the
head. Working surfaces for designers, architects,
artists and draughtsmen are tilted to avoid this. For
the rest of us, to avoid bending the head forward
when reading, the book or paper needs to be held up.
Rather than sitting with head bent when paperwork
such as ledgers, computer print-outs or working
drawings has to be flat on the desk, it is better to lean
forward supporting oneself on the table or desk with
the elbows.

If a lot of reading or writing has to be done, a
tilted desk saves bending the head forward. These are

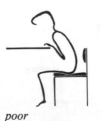

poor

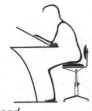

good

not widely available, but a drawing board propped up on books provides a fairly good substitute. It used to be that a ledger clerk sat on a stool or stood at a high inclined desk, the working surface tilted towards him just like the music on a musician's stand or the bible on a lectern. Yet today, outside schools, no inclined desks are in general use.

For the office worker most of whose day is spent at a desk, a comfortable position is essential. If the chair does not support the small of your back, put a little cushion there. The desk should be high enough to allow the knees to tuck right in under it and let you sit fairly upright to write on it but should not be so high that it is uncomfortable for the arms and shoulders; in other words, not much above elbow height when sitting relaxed.

Copy typists risk postural stress by repeatedly looking down at one side or the other to copy from the paper or notepad on the desk. This could be avoided if the material to be copied were put up higher—for instance, on an inclined clipboard or propped up behind the typewriter.

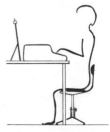

Typing imposes a fair amount of strain on the back, particularly the neck and upper back, and on the shoulders, because a typist often has to sit with arms unsupported for quite some time. The typewriter should be at a height that allows the upper arms to hang relaxed with only the weight of the forearms having to be lifted. A typist should sit as near to her typewriter as possible without this cramping her movements. If she sits too far back from the typewriter, she has to lift the whole arm forward to reach, increasing the strain put on the upper back.

Whereas a housewife should vary her posture by trying to do some jobs sitting down, the office worker should get up and walk about when possible.

—in a car

Driving is another activity which gives a lot of people a lot of backache even if they are otherwise free of back trouble. So it is important that the sitting posture is as good as possible.

The trouble is basically that the driver is working in a flexed posture and the effects are made much worse by any deficiencies in the design and construction of the seat itself. The commonest criticisms of car seats reported in *Motoring Which?* are lack of lumbar support, absence of lateral support and lack of thigh support. The first two are faults in the design of the seat itself and the last is partly a matter of inadequate seat length.

Adjust the car seat and angle of the back rest so that the pedals and the gear lever and steering wheel can be comfortably reached. When the driver's knees

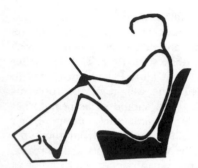

poor seat for tall driver: no lumbar support, little leg room, seat too low

are bent up too high because the seat will not go back far enough, the remedy may be to have the seat raised on blocks—provided this can be done securely and there is enough headroom. In some cars, the runners of the seat can be moved so that you have more backward or forward positions. Before you make alterations to your car's seat, check that this will not interfere with your vision and control: the seat, however poor, was designed with the visual and control aspects of driving that car in mind and if altered, proper vision and hand and foot control may be affected.

Backache from car driving is partly a postural stress but some of it comes from the movements of the car transmitted to the driver.

A car's seat should never be so springy that you bounce more than it does and the padding should give lateral support to prevent being thrown sideways on cornering, otherwise the spine is unsupported and can become twisted. If there is not enough lumbar support, use a cushion or anything that gives support in the small of the back. However, it is better not to use an inflatable cushion: this would aggravate the problem of lack of sideways control because on cornering and pressing on pedals, air in the cushion will move to the 'wrong' side and this would tend to force the body into an even worse lateral displacement.

There are numerous aids to seat comfort sold in car accessory shops Anything that supports your low back and prevents it from flexing, or gives added sideways support may help. Another solution is to have a back rest made individually moulded to fit you in any seat, but you must be able to fix it securely to the car seat—ask the supplier about this. Remember, however, that anything inserted for seat comfort occupies space and reduces the effective length of the seat. A good, though expensive, solution is to install a new seat of the kind used by rally drivers, which supports the back all round and is adjustable—but try it out before you buy.

While driving, you scarcely change your position and your range of movement is restricted by the position of the hand and foot controls. Try to be relaxed while driving—and that is not easy if you are an aggressive, anxious driver or if you cannot see properly because of dirty windows or badly adjusted mirrors. To help prevent tenseness and stiffness in the neck, whenever you have to stop—for instance, at lights or hold-ups—move the neck about a bit: shrug your shoulders a few times, raising them as high as possible towards your ears and then suddenly drop them.

It helps on a long journey to stop and take a little exercise at frequent intervals. Taking a short walk, even just around the car, provides a change of position and therefore movement of the back. When stopping for petrol, always get out of the car.

When driving in difficult conditions, such as fog or heavy traffic, one tends to lean forward towards the windscreen, holding the body away from the seat by pulling on the steering wheel. If these conditions are prolonged, it would be less tiring to adjust the seat into a more upright position or move the whole seat forward one notch.

relaxed driving position with good lumbar support and adequate seat height

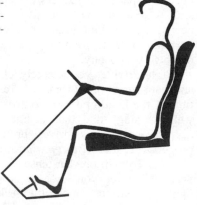

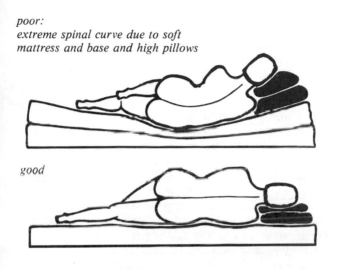

poor:
extreme spinal curve due to soft
mattress and base and high pillows

good

lying in bed
Provided your back does not bother you and you
wake without giving it a thought, it does not matter
whether you sleep in a haystack or a hammock, or in
the expensive oblivion of the most luxurious bed ima-
ginable. However, many people with chronic back
trouble find that soft or sagging mattresses are bad
for them, and some who never normally suffer from
their back find that a soft bed leaves them stiff in the
morning. A good bed supports the body evenly, not
allowing the buttocks to sink too deeply, and is easy
to move on, requiring little effort to change position.

When buying a bed, choose a reasonably firm mattress. It is better to buy one which feels too hard

rather than too soft. If it is too hard on the surface, this can be overcome by putting an extra blanket under the sheet. Avoid buying a bed with a base which is soft and springy; good mattresses are best on a firm or solid base.

The so-called orthopaedic or posture mattresses which contain their own stiffening are expensive because of the extra stiffening, and limited sales. A disadvantage is that they are heavy and do not bend like ordinary mattresses, and you may therefore need to get someone else's help to turn it. Some people who have bought such a bed found that it aggravated their back trouble. Do not be pressurised into buying one by persuasive sales techniques.

If your bed is soft and beginning to sag, putting a board under the mattress helps to counteract this— but not if the mattress itself is giving with age. The board should be as wide as the width of the bed and in length at least as long as the distance from your head to your buttocks.

When you are away from home, if you are worried by the softness of strange beds, put a cushion or pillow under the middle of the mattress. Some hotels will provide a board to go under a mattress, on request. Or you can buy a hinged fibreglass board which folds flat to go into a suitcase—but it is rather expensive.

For most people, it is better to sleep with only one pillow, and not too thick a one at that, placed between the head and shoulders to support the neck rather than the head. For someone who sleeps mainly on his side, particularly someone with broad shoulders, two pillows or one fat one would probably be more comfortable.

The main thing to avoid is too many pillows or too thick a pillow. This pushes the head up, stretching the neck, and while asleep the neck is then apt to bend sideways or forwards and the spine become flexed. Another bad situation is when pillows get under the shoulders so that the neck is left unsupported between head and shoulders.

Some people need lots of pillows at night because they have a bad chest or because their neck is too uncomfortable to lie flat. If so, it is best to organise the support so that the whole spine is supported on an incline: do it with pillows if you think you can, or incline the whole bed up by putting the legs at the head end up on blocks. The aim is to keep the whole spine, trunk and head in the neutral position. Normally, people regularly change their sleeping posture through the night. But if you have a bad neck, it is better not to make a habit of sleeping on your stomach with the head twisted to one side.

If you tend to waken with a neck which feels worse than it did the night before, you have to find some method of preventing yourself getting into extreme positions. Lying on your back with the head resting on a butterfly pillow supports the head and stops it lolling from side to side. (You can make a butterfly pillow by taking a thin or loosely filled pillow and shaking down to each end, then twisting the pillow in the centre or tying it in half.) You may find it necessary to place another pillow underneath. Simply tying a towel round your neck may also do the trick.

Everyday activities
If you can get into the habit of avoiding misuse of
your back during everyday activities, you may well
be able to prevent an acute attack from happening or
chronic backache from developing.

lifting and carrying
Injuries can be caused by a slip or fall, by twisting
and rotary stresses. They are caused by the unexpected: the box which was full when it was thought to
be empty, mistiming of the two-man lift, the load
which was stuck and you did not know it. The secret
of safe lifting is to avoid static heaving and to use
your body weight. You should always try to:

—anticipate
First, size up the job. In other words, think before
you move: how heavy is the object? is it free and not
stuck? can levers be used to reduce the stress? is the
floor space clear for you to move about without kick-
ing or stumbling over an obstruction? is the floor
slippery? where are you going to put the object?
where will you grasp it? is it a two-man job? (a load
shared is a load halved).

—dress for the job
For some jobs, wearing the wrong clothes makes it
more difficult. For example, do not wear clean clothes
for a dirty job so that it has to be done at arms'
length. Do not wear a long overall or coat that you
could tread on when crouching down. A tight skirt or
tight trousers prevent you bending your knees or lift-

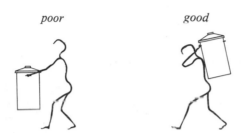

poor   *good*

ing a load between them. Watch out for bits and pieces like buttons and buckles and folds or flaps of clothing which could catch on things. Do not wear shoes that make you less stable instead of ones that grip the ground and in which you can stride or squat.

—stand properly
When you lift or shift an object, get as close to it as possible, with your feet around it rather than to one side or behind it. Put your feet so that you are firmly balanced, one foot ahead of the other, ready to move off in the right direction.

—keep a straight back
Do not tackle lifting jobs with your back rotated, twisted or bent sideways. Your shoulders and pelvis should be faced in the same direction. The danger lies in those jobs where, for instance, you try to heave something across you or turn round to jerk at a handle behind you, when you cannot use your arms symmetrically.

—get a good grip
Bend the hips and knees until the object can be reached. Grasp the object firmly. If there is nothing on the load by which to hold it, use a sling or ropes.

when lifting, hold the load close to your body to reduce the horizontal distance between lumbar vertebrae and load

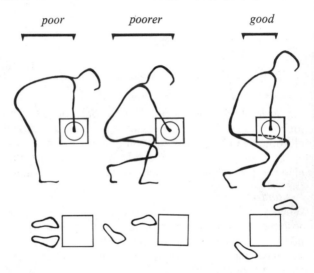

poor   poorer   good

—*keep the load close to your body*

Lifting, heaving or carrying with arms outstretched throws needless strain on the chest, upper back and shoulders. The shorter the lever, the smaller is the effort required so the closer one can get to the object, the better. A weight held out at arms' length causes as much stress on the spine as ten times that weight held at the side. The farther from your body you hold it, the greater the stress—hence the risk when lifting a box out of a car boot. Whatever you are lifting or carrying, keep its centre of gravity as near as you can over or under your own centre of gravity. This means

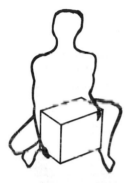

that you have to keep your knees apart enough to keep the load close to you and must use your leg muscles to help lift. Before you actually lift, it is a good idea actively to set your back muscles, then raise your head, tuck your chin in and straighten up.

—use your weight

Using your body weight can help to move things and saves the stress of direct muscular effort. If you move the body to give it momentum, it has what is called kinetic energy, and you can transfer that energy to something else. Just as you can give a cricket ball movement and thus kinetic energy enough to break a window, the body can be used in such a way that energy can be transferred to the load you wish to shift. In this way, stress on the spine can be reduced.

If not too bulky, a load can be swung horizontally, to give it kinetic energy so that its momentum can be used to swing it up to the height you want. This saves a direct lift—but it needs practice and skill.

—avoid unnecessary effort
When dealing with something large and heavy, lift it first at one end only, and get it on to a higher level before you take the full load. This halves the stress.

When lifting something with one hand, put the free hand on a table, chair or bench, to transfer some of the stress away from your back. For a job below knee level, letting one hand or elbow take the weight on the knee saves most of the spinal stress. But for a two-handed job, it is best to kneel down to it; if necessary, kneel on a hassock or wear knee pads.

Rather than carrying a heavy load, pull it on a trolley or, if that is not possible, divide it into two smaller loads, one for each hand—or a second journey, if need be.

Other parts of the body apart from the hands can be used for carrying things, which often makes the job that much lighter and easier. Using the crook of your elbow rather than your hand for holding and lifting reduces the leverage. Take the weight direct on to your thigh or pelvis, or, if you can, your shoulder, and save your spine. Use any method you can manage to avoid putting stress on your spine.

If you want to be able to lift safely and continue to do so, the more regularly you do it, the easier it is and the less likelihood of injury. It is no use trying to use your knees to save your back if you are too weak to squat on your knees. If your back is giving trouble and you have been told to save it by using your knees, start to practise to get your muscles trained for the job.

When putting things down, if you cannot safely drop the object (which is the best way), put the lifting drill into reverse. Keep the object close to your body, watch your fingers and put one end or corner down first.

in the office
In offices, risk of stress may come from carrying a stack of files or papers which has to be clutched as best one can—with the added problem of preventing items slipping out of one's grasp. Hold any such load firmly to your body so that the centres of gravity of your trunk and the load are close; use your knees when setting it down. Better still, have a sling bag or a trolley for carrying papers.

When having to bend down or stretch up for items on shelves, in the backs of drawers and on the tops of cabinets, it helps to be suitably dressed so that it is not awkward to kneel, or bend at the knees, or use a stepladder.

Also, typewriters and other desk machines sometimes have to be moved. Such a machine is heavier at the back than in front, so push it to the back of the desk and go round there to pick it up, holding it firmly against your pelvis or stomach to ease the load on arms and back.

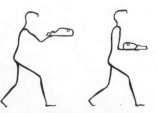

poor   *good babies and young children*

Lifting an active child who catches his legs in the side of the cot just as you are bent over to pick him up, lifting the child who has hidden behind a chair in the corner when you are in a hurry to go out shopping or get him into bed, heaving the child in and out of the bath—the stress on the back can be very great. It is partly a matter of being dressed for the job so that you can use your knees and hold the child close to your own centre of gravity. It is partly a matter of having the space so that you can use your legs and body weight. Mostly, it is a matter of pausing long enough to think out the least stressful way. If you make a habit of that, you are then less likely to strain yourself when in a hurry. If you can hold the baby with one arm, taking the weight partly on one hip, this saves the spine and leaves a hand free to support yourself. But it may not do if the child is struggling.

A cot with a drop-side makes it easier to lift the child in and out; choose a cot high enough to avoid having to stoop.

A mother can carry a young child on her hip. The father, whose hips are not as wide, may prefer to use his shoulders. Either way brings the child's weight as close to the parent's body as possible, so reducing the amount of effort required. But for someone who has a bad neck, carrying a child (or any other load) across the neck can be risky. Because of the dangers of slipping, do not carry a child in this way unless you are on level ground and able to look around with the child up there.

With a rucksack type of baby carrier where the

child is situated behind the parent, its weight is taken through the shoulders and across the back of the hips. If possible, get someone to lift it on for you, or find a safe place to prop it and the baby while you get it on to your shoulders. (A *Which?* report on baby carriers was published in March 1975.)

When bathing a small baby in a baby bath, put it on a table where you can stand or sit without stooping. When dressing a child, put him on a chair or bed to avoid undue bending. When doing up shoe laces, put the foot up on to a box or chair.

If you have to pick up a carrycot from the floor with the baby in it, get someone to help you to lift it, or do it from the side with knees bent. Do not lean forward and jerk it up in front of you with straight arms: this places enormous leverage on your back.

When lifting a toddler, bend your knees and go down to him and lift him close to you. Swinging a child up at arms' length can be a cause of acute back trouble. Try to avoid situations where you have to pick a rebellious child off the floor and lug him upstairs.

housework
With any household job, it is the length of time spent in any one position, as well as the effort imposed on the back, that counts. It is a good idea to change jobs (and therefore positions) fairly often as well as doing them in the way that imposes least strain on the back. Any activity where repetitive bending is required may cause trouble, particularly if it becomes fatiguing. It is not always necessary to do one job until the bitter

end when, with a little thought and organisation, it may be possible to alternate it with another. For example, instead of spending all monday afternoon standing up ironing, leave half of it until later on and do another job meanwhile.

—bed making
Making beds is a job that often makes painful backs worse, and in some cases even induces back trouble, because it requires a fair amount of effort and bending and stretching. A housewife with a bad back should persuade the rest of the family to make their own beds. Perhaps one of them would also take on the chore of making hers.

Bed making is not much of a problem where the bed is high enough for the mattress to be at hip height, narrow enough for you to reach across easily, and where you can walk all round unobstructed by walls, bedside tables and chairs. If this is impossible, have the bed on easily running castors. The old-fashioned high bedstead requires less effort to make than a low divan bed.

When making the bed, get close to it and bend at the hips and knees, keeping your back upright. If you have backache, you may find it less uncomfortable to kneel down when tucking in the bedclothes. An alternative for someone with chronic backache is to raise a low bed by putting blocks under the legs to get it to a better height.

A fitted bottom sheet and a duvet do away with the need to bend to tuck in bedclothes. When changing a fitted sheet, kneel close to the corners of the bed in turn when putting it on to the mattress. For changing pillowcases when you have a bad back, sit down.

A mattress that has to be turned should have handles fitted to the sides (and at the ends, too, if it is to be turned fore and aft). Grasp the handles and lift the side of the mattress so that you stand erect; then raise it high enough to turn it over by standing on the base of the bed; use your body weight to pull the mattress towards you and then let it fall over to the other side.

—cleaning the bath
Bending over to clean the bath puts considerable strain on the back, and this job can be done much more easily from the kneeling position. Kneel beside the bath if the layout of the bathroom permits this, and lean across the edge to reach the other side. An alternative is to sit on a chair alongside. Using a long-handled sponge or mop will minimise bending. A bath is cleaned more easily when still warm immediately after use, so keep the cleansing materials at hand— and, with luck, the others in the household will take the hint.

—cleaning the floor
Whenever possible, use a long-handled implement, such as a mop, for cleaning the floor. With a vacuum cleaner, make sure that the handle is long enough for you. Some cylinder cleaners have extension pieces and fitting one of these may help. When vacuuming, use your legs and your body weight to do the work. Above all, do not just stand and make your arms do the work: that way is bound to stress your back.

Similarly, when using a mop, carpet sweeper or broom, move the whole body forwards and backwards with the sweeping action, not just bending from the waist to get the increased reach.

Instead of vacuuming the whole house in one go, do a room or two at a time.

—cleaning windows

With any job that would entail stretching up for any length of time, it is better to bring the job down to you, if possible, or climb up to its level. When cleaning windows, therefore, stand on a chair or step-ladder, so that you can do the job without having to stretch. Or use a long-handled window-cleaning mop.

in the kitchen

The main thing about kitchen work is to plan it. First, have all the things you use regularly at hand— for instance, saucepans on the wall, plates and dishes at waist height. But there are limits to how much you can keep in convenient places. Many things have to be stowed either below thigh height in low cupboards or out of easy reach above chest height. Priorities should be on the basis of how often an article is used and how heavy it is. Ideally, heavy equipment such as a food mixer or cast iron casserole should be kept where it need not be lifted to be got out.

Whenever you have to do anything at floor level, go right down to it. Bend your knees to lift dishes in and out of the oven. When lifting a heavy casserole, hold it close to your body with your elbows bent. To save your back, you could put a stool at the side of

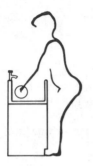

poor working posture: sink too low, no room for feet

the oven, squat down, put the casserole on the stool, re-position the body and lift the casserole on to the top of the cooker or working surface.

Having a tall stool in the kitchen is a good idea so that you can alternate between sitting and standing. A stool should have a footrail and needs to be of a height to suit the height of the working surface.

The height of working surfaces—sink, draining board, table or working area—matters a great deal to postural stress. The correct height varies with the job being done as well as from person to person. The surface should be high enough so that the housewife does not have to bend forwards, but not so high that she has to hunch her shoulders in order to do the job. A cooker or a kitchen unit can be raised by being put on a plinth. If you are too tall for washing up without stooping over the sink, raise the washing-up bowl by putting it on a small wooden stand, or on top of another upturned bowl. Someone for whom a surface is too high should stand on a small step (made out of an inverted box, perhaps) while working there. The top of a sink should be at about elbow height but work surfaces and the top of a cooker should be two or three inches lower: for a small woman, this could be 33 inches (about 85 cm), for a tall person perhaps 45 inches (about 115 cm).

What is equally important is how close you can stand to the work surface. The base of some kitchen units has a small inset which gives space for the toes underneath and enables you to get closer in. There should be a cut-out section with enough space for the leading foot below the place where the hands are busy and to allow the pelvis to rest against the sink. This is impossible where the cupboards fit vertically below the leading edge of the sink or work top. An open space under a work top would allow you to sit while working there.

washing hair and shaving
Leaning forward over a dressing-table or washbasin to see in a mirror is a frequent cause of backache. It can be avoided by bringing the mirror nearer, either putting it on an extension arm or fixed on the wall beside the basin. While shaving, the fact that your arms are raised increases the work load on the back if you have to bend forward. For arranging one's hair, the mirror need not be so close, but must be at a suitable height. For a tall person who would have to stoop to see in the mirror over a washbasin, raise the mirror farther up the wall. Better still, have a large dressing-table mirror with a comfortable chair in front.

Bending over a basin to wash one's hair puts undue stress on both the neck and the back. It may help to sit on a stool and rest your elbows on the side of the basin or sink. A better way is to wash the hair under a shower in the bath. You can buy a cheap shower attachment to fit on to the taps.

doing the washing
When washing by hand, do not use a sink or basin that makes you stoop: it is better to put a bowl at the right height for you in the sink or on the draining board.

The main problem with washing is that wet clothes and bed linen are much heavier than dry ones. Lifting wet sheets and towels in and out of a low washing machine is the sort of movement that might eventually cause back trouble. When taking clothes out of a washing machine, a low chair or stool beside the machine makes a good point of transfer. Try to make sure that you lift only one piece of wet washing at a time. If transferring something heavy like a large wet bath-towel to the spin drier of a twin-tub machine, do it one end at a time.

To take the wet clothes out to hang them up, use a basket on wheels if you have one. When hanging up the washing, have the line within easy reach so that you do not have to stretch to it. A pulley or clothes prop can be used to make it higher once it is full. Keep the pegs, too, close at hand and put the washing basket on a stool or chair so that you do not have to bend down needlessly.

—ironing

As with any working area, an ironing surface should be high enough to avoid stooping, yet low enough to allow the arms to function without raising the shoulders. If the surface is too high, the arm muscles are required to hold the elbow flexed instead of being locked straight and this needs more effort. Most ironing boards are adjustable, which means that one can obtain a reasonably correct height for the job, but none goes above 36 inches (about 90 cm), so a board that hinges from the wall at the right height for you may be the answer. (A report on ironing board heights was published in *Which?* May 1973.)

To iron, you should stand as close to the board or table as possible, with one foot slightly forward (this requires less effort than standing back from the board or table with the feet together). Use your body weight and sway from one foot to the other as you move the iron sideways over the material. Keep the things needing to be ironed on a stool at the side of the board to save bending.

If a lot of ironing is to be done, it is a good idea to sit down at least to some of it. This is easiest to manage with a fairly high stool or chair. Alter the height of the board to relate to your sitting position. It is important not to have it too high because having the arms continually raised imposes strain on the shoulders, neck and upper back.

poor   *good*

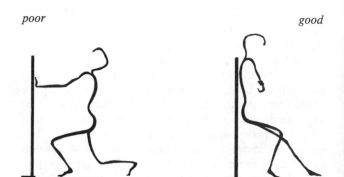

moving furniture

Few people are in training for furniture moving, so it needs to be tackled with caution if a bad back is not to follow. Do not ever attempt to shift a heavy cupboard or chest by yourself. If furniture has to be moved, try to get help. You may have to unload every single item from the cupboard on to a convenient table before you can move the cupboard—laborious but safer.

When pushing or pulling, make use of your legs and body weight. If the object to be moved is high and stable enough, you may be able to move it by leaning your back against it and pushing with your legs (wear shoes that grip the floor).

Ideally, all heavy pieces of furniture should have castors fitted on them to make them easy to move. Even with castors, the weight of a very heavy object, such as a piano, will have left a depression in the floor or carpet and the object will need to be lifted clear, for which you should get help.

carrying luggage

Suitcases and holdalls can be troublesome to someone liable to back pain, and you may not be lucky enough to find a porter or others willing to help when you are travelling. The logical solution to carrying luggage with a degree of independence is to divide the load into three: in a rucksack over your shoulders and one small case in each hand.

A suitcase with its own inbuilt castors can take much of the lifting out of moving luggage. It is possible to buy various gadgets that strap castors on to an existing suitcase. Make sure that the handle is at a comfortable height, otherwise trying to wheel a small suitcase with castors underneath would mean walking with an awkwardly twisted spine. And unless the wheels are fairly big, you will have to lift the suitcase up every step and over every kerb instead of rolling it.

Pack a suitcase downstairs to avoid having to lug it down the stairs when it is full and heavy. When travelling by car, there is the problem of loading it. Most car boots have high sills to hump the luggage over, and this imposes a major stress—especially when having to duck under the lid of the boot. If the floor of the boot is lower than the edge of the boot opening, limit the weight of individual bits of luggage so that they can be easily held in one hand, swung up to rest on the sill of the boot, then lowered with one hand while you support yourself with the other hand. Keep the floor of the boot clear of clutter so that the suitcases can easily be pushed into position. Avoid trying to push things sideways. If you can move your feet so that you pull things into place rather than having to twist your body to heave them about, so much the better.

moving an invalid
If you have to look after an invalid or disabled person, try to avoid any direct lifting, and concentrate your efforts on keeping the person balanced while moving him or her. Whenever possible, slide the person: from one end or side of the bed to the other, from bed to chair or commode. The principle to aim at is that every surface on which the invalid sits or lies should be at the same height. The transfer from one to the other can then be made easily by bridging the two with a formica-topped board and sliding the person seated on a wide sliding pad fitted with handles.

When someone has to spend most of the time in bed, it is much easier to look after him or her and to carry out any nursing duty if you do not have to bend too low. A bed can usually be raised quite easily with bed blocks. (A high bed may mean providing a step for the invalid to get out and in.) It is convenient to have a cantilever bed table which can carry books, a radio, a drink or work of any kind, but which can be wheeled out of the way so that you can get close to the head of the bed without stretching across a clutter of things.

Where lifting is a major problem, a hoist may be the answer. Small hoists suitable for use in the home are now available commercially, and you might manage to get one through your local authority social services department. If you get a hoist, make sure that either the manufacturer or a therapist teaches you how to use the hoist and its slings correctly and how to carry the disabled person at the best angle.

—moving an unconscious person

You need great skill and strength to lift an unconscious man. So, after an accident, do not move a casualty unless the place you find him in is dangerous because of fire, a flood or some other oncoming disaster. Leave everything, if you can, to a trained person, such as the ambulanceman and concentrate on essentials like keeping the casualty breathing, stopping blood loss, preventing heat loss. If there is no alternative to moving the victim, it is safer to pull him along the ground, and probably quicker unless you have help. Once the casualty is in a safe place, loosen tight clothing and roll him over on to his stomach with his face turned to one side. A warning, however: if the person is unconscious, be careful not to flex his neck when handling him because if there is a spinal injury or fracture, you could make it very much worse.

Gardening

The same rules apply to gardening jobs· as to house-hold ones: lift and carry carefully, using your legs and body weight; work upright whenever practicable; do not do too much at once, and change tasks often; get help when necessary.

The backache of gardening comes from stooping; digging; heaving lawnmower, wheelbarrow and sacks of fertiliser about the garden; hoeing, raking and sweeping. Changing the hand that does the work shares the strain on muscles.

Avoid prolonged bending and stooping by kneeling down or using a long-handled implement to do the job whenever possible. A problem with long-handled garden tools is that many of them are used by pulling them through the soil or the grass towards you and this adds to stress on the back if you are leaning forwards.

For pruning and fruit picking, there are a number of long-handled implements which allow one to avoid reaching high up above. When a ladder or stepladder is inescapable, move the ladder often to avoid over-reaching. Before you buy a ladder, make sure that you can lift and carry it without effort, and that when erected it is stable. (A report on extension ladders appeared in *Handyman Which?* February 1975.)

avoid prolonged bending . . . .

Whatever implement you use. ensure that it is of a convenient height and that it is strong enough for the job—and for you to lean on while considering the next task. The thing to avoid is any sweeping action across the body (unless it is nicely symmetrical, such as scything). It needs a good deal of work from the muscles of the trunk, and unless they are in working trim, your back may be strained. The secret is foot position, so that every action is a use of balanced body weight. Where space is too cramped, you may do better by getting down on hands and knees.

Kneeling is a very sensible posture for many jobs in the garden. Rubber knee pads are useful for wet ground and to cushion the hardness. For the more disabled, a kneeling platform can be a boon: a padded surface about four inches above the ground on a frame with handles. For those who can neither stoop nor kneel or squat, raised borders for flowers or a greenhouse with shelves would be the only possible outlets. (*The easy path to gardening*, a book intended for people who because of disability or age can no longer garden in the way they used to. is available from the Disabled Living Foundation. 346 Kensington High Street. London W14 8NS.)

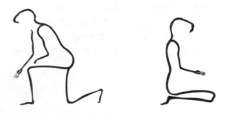

Digging is a traditional back-breaker for those untrained to it. Do not attempt to dig too much at one time. Stand over the job and try not to overload the fork or spade. Spades come in many sizes and there is no need to have a big one. You can buy a semi-automatic spade with levers which lift and turn the sod for you. Once you get the knack, it makes straightforward digging easy. Before you decide to buy one, see one in action.

A report on spades in *Which?* April 1969 included hints on

how to dig

—use the spade as a lever; raise the soil only far enough to turn it over as smoothly as possible

—cut the 'spit' (the soil to be dug each time) at the sides; use your foot to press the spade in vertically; pull the grip back towards you to break the spit free

—raise the soil by holding the shaft of the spade near its base, and do not pick up too much at a time

—grip the spade only tightly enough to control it, and do not try to work too fast.

When shovelling earth or sand, try to move the whole body weight forward, pushing with the inside of your thigh to bring the shovel under the load. Then get well forward on your legs for the actual lift. Have the job planned so that you can give each shovelful a good horizontal swing to minimise the direct lift.

when shovelling, use your legs, the inside of your knee and your body weight

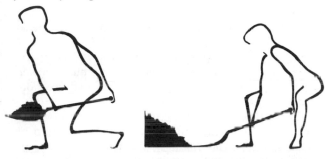

Wheelbarrows are ergonomically less satisfactory than some two-wheel trucks or garden carts. But if you have to make use of a wheelbarrow, do not overload it. It is better to make two journeys with small loads than to struggle with one. A wheelbarrow puts considerable stress on the spine because it has to be lifted and at the same time pushed—all very well if the ground is hard and level but a great effort when the ground is soft and steep. Major stresses can fall on one hand, and thus one side of the spine, if the load is high and heavy. Be sure to lift it correctly: stand between the shafts, bending at the hips and knees to reach the handles, then straighten at the hips and knees, lean forwards with your body weight—and move off.

The stress can also be great when emptying a barrow. So much so that it may be a good thing to empty it piecemeal, as filled, rather than tipping the contents out.

—mowing the lawn

Lawnmowers are heavy yet have to be heaved backwards, humped over lawn edges and in and out of sheds. Pushed mowers are the lightest and comparatively easy to manoeuvre. When using a push mower, wear boots or shoes with a good grip and use your body weight to help the movements.

Of the powered mowers, the lightest are those with electric motors which run off the mains, followed by those with petrol engines; the heaviest, weighing nearly 100 lb, are electric mowers which run off accumulators. Cylinder mowers are on the whole heavier than rotary mowers, but, being more compact, are easier to manoeuvre. Rotary mowers are handy for rough grass but there the effort of manoeuvring is far greater, particularly if the mower has small wheels.

The flatter the lawn and the simpler the shape, the less effort it is to mow. The more awkward little bits there are to mow round, the greater the total spinal stress for the area cut. For small steep slopes, it would be better to use a small lightweight machine. Even for a large area of lawn, the extra number of runs needed with a small machine may not be so very much compared with the effort of manoeuvring a big heavy machine in and out of its shed and over edges and paths.

With a motor mower, be careful when pulling the starter cord. Pulling it involves a twisting action of the spine but you can minimise this by holding the machine and pulling against the other hand. And if the cord is long enough for you to be in the right place for preventing the machine from stalling after it has started, so much the better. Do not hesitate to put an extra length on the cord. Few mowers have a kick start like a motor cycle, more's the pity—an electric starter would be even better.

Many people empty the grass box into a wheelbarrow but unless you have an ergonomically satisfactory barrow or cart, it may be easier to empty the grass box on to a sheet with handles at the corners which is easy to pull across the lawn to the compost tip.

With mowing, as with all gardening and other heavy work, the rule is not to do too much at a time. If your back starts hurting, do not struggle on to finish because the weather is right or you are going away tomorrow—stop.

if the starter cord is not long enough . . .

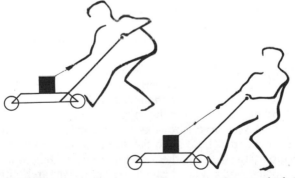

. . . fit one which is

Back pain can be due to disease in almost any of the organs in the chest, abdomen or pelvis; it can also be due to infections or growths in the spine itself. There is any number of possible causes. The symptoms come much more often not from serious disease, but from one of the mechanical derangements which afflict the spine, particularly in the lumbar region.

The spine

The spine is divided into five main regions:
    in the neck, the cervical region
    at the back of the chest, the thoracic region
    in the low back, the lumbar region
    at the back of the hip bones, the sacral region
    and below that the rudimentary tail, the coccyx.

the bones

The 7 cervical, 12 thoracic, 5 lumbar vertebrae are all separate bones of different sizes. The sacrum is a wedge-shaped and curved bone between the hip bones (at the back of the pelvis) and is made up of 5 sacral vertebrae fused together. Below the sacrum are 3 to 5 coccygeal vertebrae, either separate or fused, forming the coccyx—the remnants of a tail.

The 24 separate vertebrae above the sacrum have some features in common although they differ in shape and size. With the exception of the first two cervical vertebrae (the atlas and the axis), a vertebra has a rounded body with flat surfaces on the top and bottom; the rest of the vertebra projects backwards from the body and is called the arch. The arch consists of two bony struts called pedicles which join it to the body, two projections of bone referred to as transverse processes sticking out sideways and, above and below, two pairs of articular processes with cartilaginous joint facets. The one part of the vertebra which you can see and feel below the skin (most easily when bent forward) is the projection at the back of the arch called the spinous process. The bony layers between the spinous process and the rest of the arch are called the laminae, one on each side.

lumbar vertebra

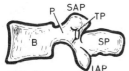

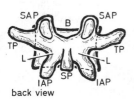

side view   view from above

back view

P	Pedicle
SP	Spinous process
SAP	Superior articular process/facet
TP	Transverse process
IAP	Inferior articular process
B	Body
C	Spinal canal
L	Lamina

joints

Each of the 24 separate vertebrae is joined above and below to its neighbour by the joints formed by the upper articular processes of one vertebra and the lower articular processes of the one above. Like the joints in the rest of the body, these have a capsule and a lining (synovium) which keeps the joint lubricated with synovial fluid.

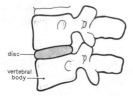

An entirely different type of joint is the joint between the bodies of the vertebrae, formed by the intervertebral disc. The disc is a very tough structure—in the healthy, tougher than the bone of the vertebral body. The centre of the disc (the nucleus pulposus) is gel-like but reinforced with strands of fibre. This is surrounded by strong criss-cross layers of fibrous tissue (the annulus fibrosus) which blend into layers of cartilage on the surfaces of the vertebral bodies. Blood supply and nerve supply do not reach the centre of the disc.

The spine has other joints, all of them synovial. For instance, the first cervical vertebra is joined to the part of the skull called the occiput by the atlanto-occipital joint, and the sacrum is joined to the parts of the hip bones known as the ilia, forming the two sacroiliac joints.

ligaments

Ligaments are bands or sheets of fibrous tissue which affect the pattern of movement taking place at a joint. They do this by providing a mechanical restraint to the direction of motion, and, by virtue of their nerve supply, relay information about the amount they have become stretched.

There is a large number of spinal ligaments, and their size and shape vary according to their parent vertebra. The main ones are the longitudinal ligaments which run down the length of the spinal column front and back, the interspinous ligaments, and the ligamentum flavum (flavum is the latin for yellow), an unusually extensible ligament which lines the back of the spinal canal, passing between the laminae of the arches.

the spinal canal

The spinal canal is formed by the backs of the vertebral bodies and discs, the pedicles, the ligamentum flavum and laminae of each arch.

Within the spinal canal lies the spinal cord and nerve roots, the most vital but not the sole content. The cord is surrounded by the cerebro-spinal fluid and is contained within a tube called the spinal dura. The space between the dural tube and the walls of the spinal canal is called the epidural space and contains a network of veins and some fatty and fibrous tissue. The dural tube extends from the base of the skull down to the sacrum. The spinal cord itself lies mainly in the cervical and thoracic regions, ending in the upper part of the lumbar region.

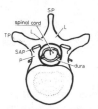

thoracic vertebra

At the sides of the spinal canal are the pedicles. Between adjacent pedicles there is a gap, the intervertebral foramen, one on each side. Arteries pass through these intervertebral foramina to supply the spinal cord, and nerve roots emerge in pairs from the spinal cord through the foramina at each vertebral level, enclosed in dural sleeves. So although the spinal dura is basically a long tube running the length of the spinal canal, pairs of dural root sleeves project from it, one on each side, where each pair of nerve roots leaves the spinal canal.

In the cervical and thoracic regions, the nerve roots emerge from the spinal cord regularly at each vertebral level. The lumbar and sacral nerve roots all emerge in a cluster from the end of the spinal cord. To the old anatomists, this cluster had the appearance of a horse's tail, so they called it the cauda equina, and it is still known as this.

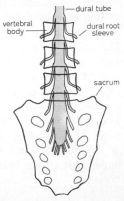

dural tube and emerging nerve roots at lumbar and sacral level

*lowest lumbar
vertebra*

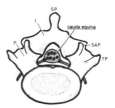

The spinal canal and its contents are protected from injury by bone and ligaments and muscle. The protection is there in all postures and throughout movement. Direct injury of the cord is rare except when the spine is fractured or dislocated, or penetrated by sharp instruments, bullets or shrapnel.

The spinal canal changes its length with spinal movement. On bending sideways, it becomes longer on one side than the other. On bending forwards and flexing the spine, the whole canal lengthens, more so behind than in front. The change in length in the cervical and lumbar regions may be as much as 25 per cent, and the contents of the spinal canal must adapt accordingly. On bending back and arching your spine, the intervertebral discs tend to bulge backwards and the ligaments lining the back of the spinal canal slacken and bulge forwards into it.

The intervertebral foramina—gaps between each vertebra—open and close considerably in the course of vertebral movement as the neighbouring vertebral arches approximate and separate. The nerve roots, particularly in the lower lumbar region, move in and out of the intervertebral foramina. This happens to some extent on sideways bending but mainly when a lower limb is stretched. If you were to lie on your back and raise one leg with the knee straight until it is vertical, the fifth lumbar or first sacral nerve root can move out of the canal by as much as one centimetre.

C

Pain

For pain to be felt, there must be a nerve supply. Nerve fibres, some of which are a metre long, connect the nerve cells in the spinal cord with nerve ends in all parts of the body.

Nerves have two main types of fibre: 'motor' fibres which convey impulses to muscles to stimulate them into activity and 'sensory' fibres which convey information via the spinal cord to the sensory cortex of the brain about touch, pressure, temperature, position and movement. If pressure is great, the temperature is high or the joint position is extreme, the sensation may be painful, but pain also arises when non-specific sensory fibres are stimulated. Pain is felt in a given part of the body either when the nerve endings are stimulated locally as a result of injury or inflammation, or when nerve fibres are irritated in their course (this occurs commonly as the sensory nerve root leaves the spinal canal). The resulting nerve impulses are not registered as pain in a given part of the body until they reach the brain.

Pain can arise from almost any of the tissues in the spine, normally with the exception of the centre of the disc and the ligamentum flavum that lines the spinal canal. In a healthy person, neither of these two tissues has a nerve supply and pain impulses do not start in them.

Back muscles are a common site for backache not only when they are fatigued by postural stress but if as a result of an injury they are sprained or undergo a minor tear. Also, when a neighbouring part of the spine is painful and inflamed, back muscles may be held taut to guard against a painful movement. This in turn may fatigue them and add a little to the pain. Occasionally, if the nerve irritability becomes intense, the muscle may go into spasm and this can be very painful.

Pain from the more superficial muscles and ligaments can be felt quite locally; from around the synovial joints, it is less clearly located, and from the surface of the intervertebral disc, it feels deep and too diffuse to tell exactly where it arises. Where the nerve fibres themselves are being irritated, pain can be felt anywhere in the region supplied by that nerve root. For instance, pain felt in the back or down the leg may arise from lumbar or sacral nerve roots.

Root involvement or nerve root lesion are the words used by doctors to indicate that something is irritating a nerve root by deforming it and putting it in tension, by compressing it or angulating it so that its blood supply is hampered. The result may be pain, and other symptoms, too. If a motor nerve root is involved, the muscle may show signs of weakness and reflexes may be affected.

Constant irritation of the nerve root and its sleeve may set up inflammation. Inflammation can lead to adhesions forming between the dural tube and the walls of the spinal canal, the surrounding ligaments and the synovial joints as well as in the intervertebral foramina. The effect is to restrict the freedom of the nerve root to slide in and out with normal movements of the spine and limbs. When adhesions are present, there is more likelihood of episodes of pain.

It is rare for all the fibres of a nerve root to be

damaged. In most cases, only a small proportion of fibres is affected.

Often, pain is felt in an area much wider than its actual site of origin, and can be felt in sites remote from the source even when there is nothing apparently wrong with the tissues where the pain is felt. This is called referred pain. The mechanism of referred pain is not fully understood. Probably it occurs when the discharge of painful impulses from the source becomes intense enough to overspill, as it were, and stimulate pain sensation in other tissues supplied by the same nerve root. When this happens, the referred pain is often accompanied by other symptoms: a feeling of dullness, heaviness, tingling and perhaps coldness. Pain felt across the back of the hips, round the groin, across the buttocks, down the thighs to the knees and even farther, may be referred from the ligaments and joints in the lumbar spine. As soon as the cause of the referred pain has been relieved, all the associated symptoms should clear.

—other symptoms

Although pain is the most typical symptom when a nerve root is irritated, it is not the only one. Muscles may be weakened, the skin of the leg and foot may become insensitive, and there are other symptoms such as pins and needles, tingling, heaviness, constriction, cramp. These are all the result of something affecting the nerve in its passage from the spine. Consider what happens when you hit your funny-bone (the bony projection on the inside of the elbow): the ulnar nerve there is rather exposed and if you bang it you can feel a shock down to the tip of your little finger and part of the ring finger, and the muscles of your hand may let go; if it is just tapped, you may feel pins and needles down to the fingers.

Another common experience is of the foot or hand going to sleep. Often, when sitting with the thigh caught on the edge of a chair, or when there has been pressure on the inside of the arm during the night, the foot or hand becomes temporarily paralysed with complete loss of all feeling and muscle power. This is due to nerve compression, or rather the result of the blood supply to the nerve being obstructed. As the nerve recovers, there are feelings of tingling, of heat or coldness, and finally of pins and needles before coming back to normal.

interpreting symptoms
There is an endless variety of symptoms of pain, altered sensation, stiffness or weakness, and symptoms are often difficult to explain. One person may be crippled with back pain and frightened to move; another may be unable to keep still and is always getting up, sitting down and fidgetting about; a third may have no back pain as such but finds that on walking his leg aches and goes weak. The significant point is that the symptoms are generally linked to the mechanical functions of the spine: pain is made better or worse by certain movements and postures and is related to the activities of the day in one way or another.

When the doctor is trying to diagnose the origin of symptoms, he has to juggle with all the relevant factors and look for features which help to localise the source of trouble. The site of pain and how far it spreads, and the factors which make it better or worse are the starting point. He has to check whether the posture of the spine is due to a deformity or is being affected by pain; similarly with spinal mobility. The doctor has to find out whether the nerve roots are involved and, if they are, whether the nerve fibres in the root are damaged. In the spinal column itself, an X-ray may reveal degenerative change in the discs or synovial joints which may or may not be the site of pain. Or it may show weaknesses and abnormalities present since birth. Just because a disc, for example, is found to be degenerated or because a minor congenital weakness is present, this is not necessarily the cause of the pain.

Mechanical factors are not all that the doctor has to take into account for his diagnosis. The problem of interpreting back symptoms is that almost every derangement in the lumbar spine has subsequently been shown to be present in a large proportion of people who have no serious back trouble. Everyone gets some wear and tear in the spine and back symptoms are common in all walks of life, but only a few people are disabled by them—and not all of these people have objective signs of damage to the nerve root. The doctor must also consider his patient's personality when interpreting the significance of pain, particularly recurring and chronic pain.

Once you have had a certain kind of pain, you are more likely to get it again. Many people develop a familiarity to pain, and take recurrences in their stride or even ignore them. For others, this is less easy and circumstances conspire to reinforce their pain so that it has an increasingly disabling effect. Partly it is a matter of individual pain tolerance, which in turn is related to physical fitness: a given pain is likely to have less effect on a physically fit person.

Pain is a subjective sensation; it cannot be measured and may vary from day to day. Apart from the local condition itself, it is affected by many factors, such as previous experience of pain, an upset in personal relationships, worry about a job, an illness or the menopause. Symptoms can become genuinely much worse when a person has other causes for anxiety, is bereaved or under financial pressure—and prolonged pain can itself be depressing.

Back injuries
Events associated with back injuries are falls, blows on the back, unskilful lifting, and strain such as heaving at something which proves to be stuck or unexpectedly heavy. Back pain can be immediate or, although you may feel that something has happened in your back, it is not until the next morning that the pain gets severe because the inflammatory reaction to the injury may take that length of time to build up.

It is difficult to say what is actually injured in such cases. It may be a muscle or a ligament. A healthy disc is unlikely to be injured because it is too tough. It is more likely that the cartilage on the surface of the vertebral body, to which the fibres of the disc are attached, will have been injured, causing microscopic cracks.

With more severe injuries, a fracture of vertebral bodies can occur, a common site being at the transitional level between the thoracic and lumbar regions where there is less mobility. Mostly, these are simple crush fractures, causing little or no deformity or trouble. Similarly, transverse processes are quite often fractured but again this causes little disability. Fractures generally become serious only if fragments compress the nerve tissues in the spinal canal or if the fracture itself leaves the spine unstable.

A fracture in the vertebral arch in the lower lumbar region is also common. This particular fracture does not occur suddenly, like breaking an arm, but develops gradually from repeated strains—it is very like the so-called 'fatigue' fracture in metals.

These fractures may occur without giving rise to much pain and, in the majority of cases, heal and do not leave the spine unstable.

Ageing and degenerative change

The likelihood of degenerative change increases with age but it is different from the normal ageing process in that ageing affects the whole spine while degeneration begins most often in a single intervertebral segment and there may be advanced degenerative change in just one site with apparently normal discs and joints above and below. It may begin in the disc itself, in the synovial joints or in ligaments—particularly the interspinous ligaments.

As one gets older, the spine tends to become stiffer. Not only is the total range of movement less with age but the tissues in the spine are stiffer in being less easily deformable; their shock-absorbing capacity is thus reduced. Also, the tissues become rather more fibrous. To some extent, similar changes occur locally during the process of degeneration. A completely degenerated intervertebral joint—disc, ligaments and joint facets—is stiff and fibrous, and it has lost height.

Degenerative change begins a good deal earlier in those who are engaged in unskilled heavy manual labour. It can also start early as a result of injurious athletic activity (but some experienced weightlifters have no more degenerative change than sedentary workers). Violent exertions and unskilled effort can, it seems, cause minor damage to the cartilage between the discs and bodies, or to the ligaments. If repetitive, there is a cumulative effect leading to degeneration even though none of the incidents themselves felt worse than a momentary jarring.

Back pain and degeneration are not invariably

associated. Plenty of people acquire major degenerative changes in their spine without ever complaining of back pain.

disc degeneration
A completely degenerated disc is narrower than normal. (On an X-ray the disc itself does not show, only the space between vertebral bodies.) As well as being narrow, it is stiff, fibrous and dry. When it reaches that state, it is unlikely to cause serious trouble. It is in the early stages of degeneration that injuries and symptoms are more likely.

The first obvious sign of degenerative change is the appearance of small ruptures in the fibrous layers surrounding the nucleus (the annulus fibrosus), through which the nucleus tends to spread. Though the healthy disc is a very strong material—stronger, in fact, than the bone of the vertebral bodies above and below it—this becomes less true with the onset of degeneration. At some stage, the disc becomes much more readily injured and this stage ends only when the stiffness and narrowing are well advanced. While it is vulnerable in this way, the person can be subject to repeated back trouble. A degenerating disc bulges more easily, particularly backwards. Mechanically, it does not restrain the shearing forces between vertebral bodies as efficiently, and therefore the ligaments and joint facets may have to resist abnormal strains. It is at this stage that some people undergo a disc prolapse. This is a major rupture or herniation of material from the nucleus of the disc through the annulus and it can cause trouble, particularly if it involves any of the nerve roots.

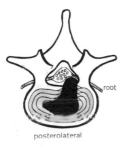

posterolateral

*prolapse trapping
nerve root*

The commonest direction for prolapse is back-wards and sideways. In a backwards and sideways prolapse, a single nerve root only is likely to be involved. But if it is backwards only, the prolapse can, depending on the size of the spinal canal, involve the cauda equina itself. This is rare but, if it happens suddenly, the resulting back and leg pain with numbness, weakness and disturbance of bowel and bladder function creates a surgical emergency.

*prolapse involving
cauda equina*

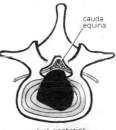

central posterior

Once the degenerative process has reached the stage of stiffness and the disc has narrowed, the risk of prolapse is reduced and the system becomes more stable once again.

The symptoms of a disc prolapse arise from the associated inflammation which is not of infective origin but is similar to the inflammation following any injury. The inflammation develops over a day or so and spreads to involve other tissues at the same level. It may cause back pain or sciatic pain, depending on whether the inflammatory change affects the tissues of the spine, the nerve root or both. Following the inflammation, some adhesions may develop between the disc and the dural tube or dural root sleeve in someone who remains immobile for too long.

It is difficult to say how much pain arises from the disc itself: certainly not from the nucleus but possibly from the outer edges of the annulus. However, with repeated damage and attempts at healing, the disc can acquire nerve endings which are not normally present, and pain may arise from them.

Often associated with disc degeneration is a thickening of the edges of the vertebral body, particularly around the lower surface. In some cases, these take the form of bony hooks (called osteophytes) which curl round the margins of the disc. Generally, they become commoner with age and increasing stiffness. Where disc prolapse and bony thickening of the vertebral body margin are present together, they may encroach on the spinal canal and intervertebral foramina, putting nerve roots at risk.

synovial joint degeneration
As with any other joint in the body, when spinal joints are subjected to abnormal wear and tear, such as repeated sprains, the cartilage lining the joint facets

becomes thinner and more fibrous and the articular processes tend to thicken where the capsule of the joint is attached. Mainly, this affects the upper articular processes so that the bony thickening takes up space in the spinal canal and in the intervertebral foramina. On an X-ray, these changes are difficult to see except when the articular processes have become generally thickened. Degenerated synovial joints can readily become the site of back pain and of pain referred over the buttock and down the thigh.

ligament degeneration
Ligaments, too, undergo degenerative changes. The interspinous ligament often begins to degenerate in people who can no longer freely bend forwards and have a permanently arched (lordotic) lumbar spine. The ligament becomes somewhat narrower and its structure disorganised by the formation of ruptures and cavities. It is a likely source of pain and local tenderness.

Degeneration also affects the ligamentum flavum (the yellow elastic ligament that lines the back of the spinal canal) particularly when the spine has become stiff and the ligament is no longer stretched normally. Then it becomes more fibrous, loses its yellow elastic function, and if nerve endings spread into it, can become a source of pain.

Diagnostic terms

Diagnostic labels are used by doctors to identify diseases. In some branches of medicine in which the diseases are well recognised and classified, one or two words are enough to convey the essentials of what is wrong. With back and sciatic pain, it is often difficult to be sure of the precise cause; whatever the diagnosis, almost all back conditions can be present without pain.

The doctor's main diagnostic task is to find out whether there is any serious disease. If not, the need for precise diagnosis depends on how incapacitating or how persistent the symptoms are. In most cases of mechanical derangement of the spine causing back pain or sciatic pain, the symptoms get better on their own and the need for accurate identification of the cause is less urgent than where surgical treatment may become necessary. When there is a possibility of irritation or damage of the nerve roots, the diagnosis should identify the site of trouble as precisely as possible, and should account for disturbances in both nervous and mechanical function.

The following, in alphabetical order, are diagnostic labels which are in use, some more commonly than others. In any individual case, one such label may not be enough because some diagnostic terms refer to structural, mechanical change and others to the secondary effects on nerve roots.

Not included are serious diseases, tumours or infections, and none of the causes of back pain of gynaecological or urological origin, nor the major congenital malformations such as spina bifida cystica.

A few conditions of rheumatological origin have been listed whose names you may hear and whose symptoms can be similar to those of mechanical derangements.

These descriptions are not intended as an aid to self-diagnosis: you would be unwise to use them for that purpose. When you have back pain or sciatic pain, leave the diagnosis to your doctor. If he tells you that the symptoms stem from a mechanical derangement of the spine, he will probably use one of the terms listed here.

ankylosing spondylitis is one of the inflammatory diseases whose cause is unknown. It affects the sacroiliac joints, and spreads upwards to the other joints of the spine, and may result in the joints becoming stiff. It may also involve the hips and other joints. Ankylosing spondylitis is not serious in most cases, but it can be painful.

arachnoiditis is inflammation of the arachnoid membrane which lines the inside of the dural tube. As a result, the membrane may thicken and proliferate, particularly round the nerve roots before they enter the dural root sleeves. It can cause either back pain or pain down the leg. It also occurs to some extent, and not necessarily causing pain, after any spinal operation or a myelogram (special X-ray).

cauda equina lesion is due to something constricting or stretching the bundle of nerve roots in the dural tube within the lumbar spinal canal. Because it involves all these roots within the canal and not one or two separate ones, it generally affects both lower limbs, and the nerves to the organs in the pelvis, so that in a few cases there may be bladder problems as well.

disc prolapse, disc herniation, prolapsed inter-vertebral disc—all mean rupture of the annulus fibrosus with extrusion of part of the nucleus through the rupture. This only occurs after disc degeneration has begun and is exceptional in a healthy disc. The commonest direction for a prolapse is backwards and sideways (posterolateral) to one side of the spinal canal towards the intervertebral foramen. A central prolapse is directed straight backwards towards the midline of the spinal canal; a lateral prolapse is directed sideways; the most rare prolapse—anterior—is directed forwards.

Disc prolapses are mainly troublesome if they interfere mechanically with the emerging nerve root in the region of the intervertebral foramen. They then stretch or angulate the root from its normal path and

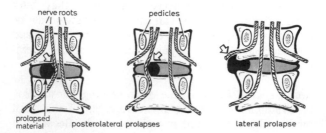

nerve roots

pedicles

prolapsed material   posterolateral prolapses   lateral prolapse

it is likely to become inflamed. In some cases, the prolapsed disc material compresses the root. This sometimes happens when there is a *sequestrated prolapse*—a prolapse of material freed from the rest of the disc which lodges in the spinal canal or in the foramen. Generally, the effect of a prolapse depends on how big it is and on how much room there is in the spinal canal and intervertebral foramen.

dural adhesions are what form, often where there has been inflammation, in the spinal canal when the dural tube becomes adherent to an old disc prolapse, or to the bony thickening round the joint facets in osteoarthrosis, and sometimes after an operation.

epidural root fibrosis is an abnormal increase of fibrous tissue round the root itself. If anything stretches the nerve root sleeve from its normal pathway or encroaches on the space it occupies in the gap between the vertebrae, the fibrous sleeve tends to thicken and become adherent to the walls of the intervertebral foramen.

fibrositis—a once-fashionable term now out of favour—was used to describe the locally painful nodules consisting of fibro-fatty cysts in muscles over the spine and buttocks.

joint fixation and *joint subluxation* are terms used to describe local stiffness of the synovial joints at one spinal level. There may be no movement at all or only a limited amount at one end of the normal range. In a few cases, the joint appears to become stuck at the extreme of the range; this may be called *subluxation* (slipping under) and it does not mean dislocation.

joint tropism is a term used by some doctors to describe an asymmetrical orientation of spinal joint facets. Normally, the two synovial joints between pairs of vertebrae are of a symmetrical shape. When they differ, and the facets face in different relative directions, movement such as rotation may be restricted and lead to greater stresses on one side than the other, or on the disc. But usually it does not cause any back trouble.

kyphosis—not a diagnosis—is a convex curvature of the spine. Kyphotic deformities are commonest in the thoracic spine but can occur elsewhere. They are seldom congenital but may be secondary to other congenital growth defects or be acquired from bad posture or be secondary to fracture or disease. Kyphosis can occur in old age due to atrophy of muscles and ligaments.

lateral root entrapment or *lateral stenosis* describes a nerve root entrapped or compressed as it emerges from the dural tube, by any mechanical derangement which encroaches on the intervertebral foramen. Prolapsed disc material may lodge in the foramen and become wedged there. As a result of disc degeneration, the margins of the vertebral bodies may thicken and become lipped, forming a bony ridge encroaching on the foramen. Similarly, as a result of synovial joint degeneration, bony thickening of the upper joint facet also encroaches on the space. The resulting symptoms are worse on bending to the affected side and bending backwards because both movements reduce the size of the intervertebral foramen.

lesion—not a diagnosis—means any morbid change in the function or texture of organs or tissues, and is used by some doctors unspecifically to refer to a change which they assume to be the cause of pain. Lesions can be present without causing pain, but are more likely to become inflamed and the source of pain than healthy tissues.

lordosis—not a diagnosis—is a concave curvature of the spine. On standing, your spine in the lumbar region is normally lordotic. An exaggerated lordosis means an unduly curved lower back.

lumbago—not a diagnosis—means pain in the lumbar region.

lumbar instability or *lumbar insufficiency* are words used unspecifically to refer to any derangement of mechanical function which causes abnormal stresses on the spine and abnormal strains in the supporting tissues. In strict orthopaedic terms, an instability is a weakness leading to deformity. A spine whose supporting muscles are weak from paralysis, pain or disuse would be unstable, and more susceptible to injury and more liable to pain from trivial strains.

lumbarisation see sacralisation.

lumbosacral strain is a term used to describe the consequences of a minor back injury or of postural stress involving the lowest lumbar disc and joints.

nipped synovial fringe is sometimes used to explain sudden onsets of back pain. In the synovial joints, there is a pad of fat in the capsule of the joint which, it is said, can get caught between the two facets. But there is no practical way of demonstrating that a nipped synovial fringe is the actual cause of pain—or that it has occurred.

osteitis condensans ilii is an increase in the density of iliac bone (upper part of the hip bone) at the lower margin of the sacroiliac joint. A disorder of unknown origin, it can cause persistent low back pain.

osteoarthrosis is a degenerative disease of joints. If it affects the spine, it is present at more than one level and in more than one region, generally the cervical and lumbar regions. It affects synovial joints and

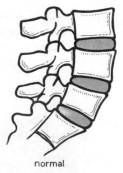
normal

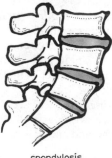
spondylosis

discs and, like any degenerative joint disease, it may be painful. It is also called *spondylosis* (and by some is called arthritis). The disease is generally accompanied by thickening of the neighbouring bone which encroaches into the spinal canal. This may then irritate the nerve roots in the spinal canal or as they emerge through the intervertebral foramina.

osteophytes are bony outgrowths or spurs forming on a bone or in fibrous tissues attached to the bone. Osteophytes may form where the tissues are under tension, partly as a result of altered patterns of movement, and are a sign of neighbouring degeneration. Osteophytes are very common: the likelihood of your getting them increases with age and stiffness. On an X-ray, they can look formidably hook-like sometimes but mostly they give no trouble at all.

osteophytosis means a proliferation of osteophytes as more than one site, usually accompanied by the general thickening of bone of degenerative joint disease. An advanced form of osteophytosis leads to a very stiff spine because the vertebral bodies become locked by the bony outgrowths. This condition is called *ankylosing vertebral hyperostosis*.

osteoporosis is a loss of bone density accompanied by a reduction in its mineral content. When this happens, and when it is severe, the spine tends to shrink in overall length so that the person becomes shorter. It is not a painful process in itself, but the joints have to adapt to the new mechanical situation and this may cause a number of episodes of arthritic pain anywhere in the spine and in the joints between the spine and the ribs. Osteoporosis leaves bone a little weaker and it may then fracture more easily. In advanced cases the vertebral bodies can collapse.

Paget's disease (*osteitis deformans*) is a bone disease of unknown cause in which the bones thicken and become more dense, and tend to deform; in the spine it may involve nerve roots and cause pain.

p.i.d.—doctors' shorthand for prolapsed intervertebral disc.

rheumatism—not a diagnosis—is a vague term used for aches and pain in muscles, bones and joints.

rheumatoid arthritis is a disease of synovial joints in any part of the body affecting the lining or capsule (the synovium) of the joint. It can affect the spine, most often in the neck, causing aching and stiffness.

sacralisation and *lumbarisation* describe minor genetic anomalies which marginally increase the likelihood of back pain. In the course of development of the spine, there are often minor variations in the level of transitions from one region to another. This is usually of no consequence, but at the lumbosacral transition when a true fifth lumbar is sacral in type and fused to the sacrum, it is called sacralised, and when a true first sacral vertebra has lumbar characteristics it is called lumbarised. Symptoms may stem from the abnormal joint which sometimes forms there or from an abnormal stress on the disc or joints at the level above.

sacroiliac strain is a term used to describe pain felt in the sacroiliac region arising from a minor injury or postural stress as a result of, for example, a lifting or twisting strain. During pregnancy, the supporting ligaments slacken as a result of biochemical changes. Normally, the ligaments tighten again after the baby is born but sacroiliac strains tend to be more likely during and after pregnancy.

sacroiliitis is inflammation of the sacroiliac joints.

sciatica—not a diagnosis—is pain felt down the thigh and leg in the area of distribution of the sciatic nerve. (The sciatic nerve supplies the buttock and back of the thigh, and all of the leg and foot.) Sciatic pain can arise when a disorder of the lumbar spine interferes mechanically with a nerve root.

scoliosis—not a diagnosis—means a sideways curvature of the spine. A postural scoliosis means such a curve in an otherwise normal spine. Someone with sciatic pain, for example, may adopt a sideways curve (sciatic scoliosis) to reduce the tension on an affected nerve root and so minimise the pain. A structural scoliosis is the result of a deformity of the spine, and can cause pain. There are a number of causes of scoliosis, not all of them understood.

slipped disc—not a diagnosis—is just a popular term used to describe a prolapsed intervertebral disc. The term is misleading because it implies something like a washer which slips in or out of place, and this is not what happens. Try to avoid it.

spondylolisthesis is a deformity of the spine due to one vertebra having slipped forward in relation to the one below it. Common sites are between the fifth lumbar vertebra and the sacrum, or between the fourth and fifth lumbar vertebrae. It is present in 5 to 6 per cent of the male population in most countries; it is less common in women. Most people are unaware that they have it, but it can cause back pain.

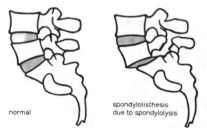

normal

spondylolisthesis
due to spondylolysis

Most commonly it arises in the neural arch and is due to a fracture (spondylolysis). The forward slip may also arise because of minor errors of growth in the vertebral arch at the fifth lumbar or first sacral level. Because of this underlying weakness, the arch may become attenuated and lengthened during the adolescent spurt of growth and the fifth lumbar vertebra slips forward over the sacrum. Parents notice a deformity of the spine and that the child's trunk is comparatively short; the child may notice some stiffness or difficulty at games. Otherwise, these children are perfectly healthy, and once the spine is fully grown, the slipping is arrested, the spine becomes more stable and there is seldom any further trouble, not even when it comes to childbearing.

Another common site for spondylolisthesis is at the synovial joints. Where there is degeneration, the damaged joints may become deformed by the stress on them. The deformation allows a small amount of forward slip between the vertebral bodies, usually at the fourth/fifth lumbar level, resulting in constriction of the intervertebral foramina and sometimes of the spinal canal itself. It happens mostly in middle-aged women. The person may have had back pain for a long time with a recent onset of more pain in the leg.

spondylolysis is a fracture in a vertebral arch, due to an injury or to 'fatigue failure' as in metals. If the defect is present on both sides, the vertebra can become unstable because the body may separate from the arch. In some cases, the defect heals spontaneously like other fractures. Some races—Eskimos, for instance—and some families are especially prone to spondylolysis. It can occur from childhood onwards, particularly in those who are athletic or go in for gymnastics. It often causes no symptoms (even professional footballers and weightlifters have had spondylolysis which has caused no interference with their sporting careers). However, spondylolysis can lead to spondylolisthesis.

stenosis means a narrowing. Spinal stenosis refers to narrowness or constriction of the spinal canal. In the established case of spinal stenosis, the cauda equina (the bundle of lumbar and sacral nerve roots within the dural tube in the spinal canal) may be compressed whenever the lumbar spine is arched backwards. In this position, the spinal canal is shorter, the soft tissues bulge into it and the space available to the cauda equina is reduced and this may restrict blood flow and the flow of cerebro-spinal fluid in the dural tube. When this leads to trouble, the legs become painful and weak: the person may find that he can walk so far and then has to sit or bend down for a while before he can go farther. Bladder trouble may also develop. The actual symptoms vary according to whether the whole cauda equina is constricted or just one or two nerve roots.

There is considerable variety in sizes of spinal canal. The overall dimensions of the canal are a relevant factor in the potential effects of bony thickening or disc prolapse on the cauda equina or nerve roots. Some people are born with a very narrow spinal canal so that only a minor change or a minor injury is needed to trigger symptoms. In others, stenosis may happen gradually over the years, the main contributory factors being osteoarthrosis where the bone surrounding the spinal canal thickens, degenerative spondylolisthesis, or a massive prolapse of disc material.

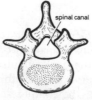

normal canal

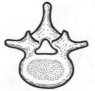

stenosis due to congenitally narrow canal

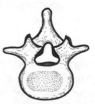

normal canal with stenosis due to bony hypertrophy and degenerative change

Everything you do or do not do during an acute episode of back pain should be directed first towards relieving the pain and then to getting back to normal activity as soon as possible. Avoid the movements and postures that cause pain, in order to relieve the painful tissues of mechanical stress and let them heal as quickly as possible.

The following advice may be useful for those who have seen their doctor during earlier episodes and been reassured that the trouble was not serious and were told to go home to rest and take a painkiller, and whose present attack is similar in all essentials to previous symptoms.

General advice on treatment cannot apply to every individual. If your doctor gives instructions that conflict directly or indirectly with what you read here, do what the doctor says and ignore this. (But if you do not get better, go back and talk to him again.)

an acute attack
The typical attack of back pain begins after exertion for which you were unfit—an afternoon's hard work in the garden on the first day of spring, for example. An attack may follow a period in which you have been getting a mild, nagging backache which you had hoped would get better by ignoring it. Or it may be a recurrence of old trouble from which you had never properly recovered: in this case, it may have needed only a trivial movement to exacerbate it—such as leaning across to open the car door on the passenger's side.

When the pain comes on, stop whatever you are

doing, even if it is just sitting. If you find yourself fixed, and unable to straighten up, get on to a couch or somewhere level so that you can remove stress from your back and relax; then steadily straighten up until you can hollow your back again. If you can do this, it may help to abort the acute attack. Someone who has had an attack before will recognise the warning signs and go and lie down. A hot bath may be comforting but there is the risk that if you lie in the bath with your back flexed, you may become completely stuck there. If you do have a bath, kneel rather than sit.

Take a painkiller if the pain prevents sleep.

You may wake the following day to find it difficult to get out of bed and that it hurts when you cough or sneeze. Do not sit up (you probably cannot) and lie still to avoid pain. When you have to get up to go to the lavatory, roll carefully out of bed and crawl there. Crawling may be less painful than trying to walk; it is when getting up from the horizontal to the vertical that pain is most likely. Be cautious when getting into a sitting position.

The worst of the pain should start to wear off in a day or so, but if the acuteness does not subside fairly quickly or you notice any peculiar signs and symptoms such as numbness, pins and needles, frequency or difficulty in passing water, weakness, dizziness, giddiness, nausea, severe referred pain (that is, pain apart from that which is actually in the back), the doctor should be consulted without delay.

The painful stage usually lasts for three or four days, and you may have to stay in bed during this time.

—*staying in bed*

The first thing to organise is a comfortable position in bed. It is important to try to rest horizontally, thereby taking the body weight and a lot of stress off the back. Being propped up is probably a bad thing, so be prepared to lie on your back or side with one or at the most two pillows. It is not essential to lie flat on one's back, and with severe back pain, you may not be able to do so. Try to get as comfortable as possible in a position that relieves the pain, making use of pillows or cushions to give support. For example, if you want to keep your spine supported, try putting either a pillow in the small of your back or a towel folded to fit under the hollow of your back. With a sagging mattress, it may be helpful to put a pillow or cushion under it to give support. Some people when they have sciatic pain find lying on their side with the affected leg uppermost on a pillow a comfortable position. Others prefer to lie on their back, either flat or with a pillow under one or both knees. Some people find lying face down to be a relief.

If you want to read, lie on your front with your head over the end of the bed and the book on a chair or on the floor; if on your back, hold the book above your face.

Although it may be possible to find a comfortable lying position, moving about from one position to another can put quite a stress on the spine unless you use your arms, so it helps to have something firm to hold on to. If you want to turn over in bed, you will need room to roll over, so start by wriggling over to one side of the bed. Then bend your knees bringing your heels up to your buttocks, fold the arm of the opposite side to which you intend to turn across your chest and, using the weight of your knees, roll, keeping your shoulders in line with your hips. A nylon bottom sheet makes turning in bed easier. For getting out of bed, come to the edge lying on your side, bend your knees up, then let the legs hang out to act as a counterweight, as you push yourself upright. But have a chair at hand to lean on when you get to your feet.

If you cannot get comfortable in bed and you think it too soft, get someone to put a board under the mattress or put the mattress on the floor. Alternatively, put a sleeping bag or a quilt on the floor with cushions to support you.

There is no need to eat or drink much: the less need you have to keep getting up to go to the lavatory during the first day or so, the better. So a minimum of food, if any, is sensible, and only as much to drink as thirst demands. You may have to lie on your front to feed yourself. Alcohol should be treated with caution; with some people it makes the pain worse, or it may interact with other drugs you are taking.

You may find that you are temporarily constipated, but there is no need to worry about this. It may be due partly to immobility, partly to the pain caused by trying to go to the lavatory. If you are taking painkillers which contain codeine, they can be constipating.

Move your legs regularly if this does not hurt. Exercises as such at this stage may not be possible. But the longer you lie absolutely still like a log, the longer you will need for recovery because you become stiff and your muscles weaken. Therefore, regularly—say, every hour—spend a few minutes moving your toes, feet, ankles, knees and hips. You may be in the most awful pain and frightened to move but somewhere a movement can be made without pain and that is the starting point. Begin with wriggling the toes, circling the ankles, working the feet up and down, flexing and extending the knees. Then start hip movements by moving the knees, one at a time, up and down and side to side. This mobilises your back without stressing it. You can do this on your back or lying on your side. If a certain movement hurts, avoid it and try to find another which does not. As an alternative, and to give the legs a rest, try slow deep breathing. Another type of movement that can usefully be tried is rhythmically to tense your muscles: set, hold firm and relax. Try the buttock muscles and the muscles on the front of your thigh first, then your abdominal muscles. Try also your hamstring muscles and the ones in your calf and foot—but be cautious about getting cramp. Do these movements for a few minutes only, every hour or so, and always before getting out of bed to go to the lavatory.

Many people get relief from the application of heat where the pain is. Probably the most effective way is to fill a plain rubber hot water bottle and wrap it inside a small bath towel wrung out in hot water. Be careful that it is not hotter than you can bear. Beware of the risk of scalding the skin, which may be less sensitive over a painful area. Start by applying it for brief spells, and then, when tolerable, keep it on firmly for about 15 minutes. Alternatively, you could use an electric pad or a radiant lamp, but not too hot or for too long.

If there is someone who can massage your back and this makes you feel better, that is fine. For instance, the feeling of warmth after rubbing in a liniment can be temporarily comforting. The effect of an ointment containing a mild rubefacient (something which makes the skin red) stems partly from the rubbing in and from the warmth it creates. But, however you have applied the heat and therefore made the skin sweat, it is as well to keep it warm afterwards.

On the other hand, some people get relief from applying something cold—such as ice cubes wrapped in a towel.

During a spell of back pain, a feeling of support is very welcome. There are plenty of simple ways of achieving this. An ordinary corset fastened as tight as possible can be excellent during an attack. Alternatively, a belt, two to six inches wide, worn round the hip bones and pulled tight, helps to provide support—something for the muscles to lean against, so to speak.

There are dozens of folk remedies and commercial preparations for backache. Provided they have no curious after-effects, do not hesitate to use them if they work for you. However, acute back pain generally gets better whatever you do, so there is no point in spending large sums of money.

Most spells of acute back pain are over the worst in 48 to 72 hours and allow the victim to be up and about in a few days. Get up for only an hour or two at a time on the first day, and then for longer each day. Dealing with shoes, trousers, socks or tights may be a problem: try, while lying on the bed or sitting on a chair, to bring your leg closer to your hand by bending sideways and flexing the hip and knee. Use any gadgets that are a help, and avoid two-handed jobs—such as doing up shoe laces (by wearing shoes that slip on using a long-handled shoe horn).

Rest frequently by lying down—on the floor, the ground or a table if you are away from your bed—not sitting. Avoid moving quickly and holding one position (including sitting) for any length of time.

Do not drive the car, and as passenger, be careful getting into one, particularly if it is parked at a high kerb. Bending the neck when getting in may bring on pain. Get in slowly or, better still, sit on the seat first and then swing the legs round and in.

Until you are 100 per cent fit again, be careful not to carry too much; if need be, resort to a trolley or a shoulder pack. Above all, do not do the movement that brought on the attack—if you know what that was. Be careful about bending and lifting and twisting movements.

—calling the doctor
If by the third day the pain in your back is not getting better and you are still immobile, ask the doctor to come. Anyway, you will need a doctor's certificate now for being off work.

The doctor when he examines you will test the movement in your legs by raising them one at a time, keeping the knees straight. This stretches the sciatic nerves. How far he can lift them without aggravating the pain is a guide to how severe the trouble is. He may try other leg movements to find out whether certain nerves are not working properly. The doctor will check whether there is any loss of sensation in any part of your body and if the reflexes are normal.

Although most back trouble is due to mechanical derangements of the spine, pain may be felt in the back arising from sources other than the spine. The doctor may therefore consider other possible causes for the pain—for instance, kidney disease, a peptic ulcer, gynaecological trouble—and give you an abdominal examination, too. Prolapse of the womb, for instance, may cause low backache which is relieved by lying down. (Although low backache of any cause may be worse before a menstrual period, a gynaecological cause for backache is not all that common.)

If the doctor decides that it is a degenerated or prolapsed disc that is causing your trouble, he will probably tell you to continue to stay in bed. Rest is prescribed to allow the associated inflammation to settle down—no other reason: discs cannot be reversed pathologically. The doctor may give you painkillers and prescribe a tranquilliser—not just to stop you worrying but because of the physical relaxation of the muscles a tranquilliser can bring. Tell him if you know that any of these upset you or which suit you. Any injection he gives you is likely to be a painkiller of some kind.

Once you have had to see your doctor or been off work, because of a spell of back pain, you are probably more liable to have to do so again than someone who has not had back trouble. This could simply be because you have broken the ice and now come to rely on the doctor. It could also suggest that the after-effects of one spell of back trouble contribute causally to the next. People who have had spells of back trouble are likely to have a stiffer spine and weaker muscles in the back and abdomen, irrespective of what caused the back trouble. It is therefore important to regain the normal mechanical and nervous functions of the spine that existed before the first attack, and good abdominal and back muscles, so as to prevent the first symptoms of back trouble from becoming chronic.

SPECIALIST EXAMINATION

If your back trouble is not better after about three weeks, or you are getting recurrent attacks of back pain, or your doctor thinks there is some other reason for your back trouble, he may suggest that you should be seen by a specialist. He can request a domiciliary visit by a consultant if he thinks you are not fit enough to go to hospital. But usually it means a visit to hospital as an outpatient to see a consultant in the orthopaedic or rheumatology or neurosurgical department. The outpatient appointment may be several weeks or even months ahead. If your case is considered urgent—on medical not social grounds—you may be seen within a few days.

In asking questions and in examining you, and in any investigations that he orders, the doctor's purpose is both to exclude the possibility of serious disease and to learn about the cause and origin of your back pain. The lengths he goes to will vary according to whether this is your first spell of back trouble or whether it is of a kind that has not responded to previous treatment. The specialist will want to know about your previous medical history, operations, severe injuries or prolonged illnesses, and whether you are having treatment at present for any other condition.

When he has completed his tests and investigations, he will have satisfied himself whether or not there is any serious disease. Do not hesitate to ask him if he has not reassured you on this point.

The first thing to say is where the pain and other symptoms are, and how far they extend; it helps to point the places out. Be prepared to go into considerable detail, when asked. The doctor will want to know how long ago the trouble began; what you were doing when, or just before, it started; what the symptoms were like to start with and how they have changed since. In other words, whether you are between attacks, in continuous pain, getting better or worse. (If by the time you see the specialist your back is better, say so; specialists are used to this. Anyway, you may want to know how to get completely well and avoid further trouble.)

You should tell the doctor what makes the pain better and what makes it worse—things like bending, sitting, walking, standing and so forth—and the effect the pain has on your usual physical activities. If you are under any strain in your work, home, relationships or other personal factors, tell the doctor in case it has any bearing on your back pain. In a few people with a mechanical derangement of the spine, emotional or psychological disturbances may interact with the back pain.

It may be difficult to describe symptoms other than pain, such as heaviness, dullness, tightness, numbness and weakness. Numbness, for example, means different things to different people. Some use it in a general way to describe a vague sensation that a leg, for instance, feels different or does not belong. But it may be taken to mean more precisely that the skin itself has lost all sensation and that you could scald it without feeling pain. Weakness, for instance, could describe a feeling of weakness due simply to pain, as distinct from weakness describing your toes dragging on the ground because you cannot bend your ankle up. Analyse the feeling or pain carefully, explain it as descriptively as you can and try to make sure that the doctor understands your meaning of the words you use.

Being able to give information about any previous back trouble before the current attack is useful. But when it is a long and complex story, it may be difficult to know how much to tell the doctor. On the whole, unless asked directly, it is better to avoid recounting in detail what has been said to you by various doctors, surgeons, chiropractors and physiotherapists you may have seen in the past. Doctors like to make their own diagnosis and it does not really help to give them other people's. The important thing is to concentrate on where the pain was and whether you had to go to bed or could continue at work; how many times you have had pain since and whether the pain then and subsequently was like it is now; whether you have had any treatment and, if so, what helped and what made it worse.

Examination
The spine will have to be examined, so be prepared to strip down to (bra and) pants with socks or tights off. The examination will hurt a bit: it is bound to because your pain is the focus of interest. Be as accurate as you can about what you feel while the doctor is examining you.

The order and extent of the doctor's examination may vary but usually it begins by an inspection of the posture of your spine because this can be affected either by symptoms or by a deformity. The range of movement and the way you do it will be looked at while you bend forwards, sideways and backwards (a few hospitals have a special device for measuring this). The doctor will move your neck and lower limbs to test for signs of increased tension in the nerve roots and will test muscle strength in the back, abdomen and lower limbs. The sensitivity of the skin on the foot, leg, thigh, buttocks is checked by touch and pinpricks; reflexes are tested at the ankle and knee and sole of the feet. And your spine will be felt for signs of tenderness, muscle spasm or deformity.

X-rays

Almost certainly you will be sent to the X-ray department either there and then or at a later appointment to have X-rays (radiographs) taken of the spine.

Before this is done, a woman should be asked about the date of her last menstrual period. There is a '10-day rule': to minimise the risk of irradiating a foetus, X-rays should be taken only during the 10 days after the beginning of a menstrual period, when there is least likelihood of pregnancy. Later, after ovulation, there may be a possibility that she has conceived and that the foetus could be affected by radiation. In some radiography departments, a man is given a thing like a cricketer's box to protect the testicles from radiation.

Generally, three or four views of the spine are taken. Sometimes, one sideways view is taken with your spine flexed fully forwards and another with it arched backwards. This can be uncomfortable, but do your best to relax and keep still so that the picture is not blurred. It is done like this in order to assess movement between these two postures at each vertebral level—whether it is absent or excessive, or abnormal in some other way.

On the film, the shadows of the bones show up in excellent detail, particularly if you are slim. It is possible to assess the size and shape of the spinal canal and its exits, which may be relevant. The discs themselves do not show, only the space available for them. (Remember this in case you happen to get a chance to look at your own pictures.)

The radiographs are seen by the consultant, and may also be seen by the radiologist—a doctor who specialises in X-ray diagnosis.

The main value of the X-rays is to confirm that there is no evidence of serious disease. X-rays can show the presence of degenerative changes in the vertebrae, and any signs of abnormalities, deformities and potential mechanical weaknesses. But do not be surprised if the doctor identifies no particular abnormality on your X-rays; this may be so even where there is an acute disc prolapse.

further tests
Depending on what has been learned so far and on how bad your symptoms are, further tests may be carried out, such as blood tests, diagnostic injections, electromyography, special X-rays. In most cases, however, it is unlikely that they will have to be done; and in any event, only some of them.

A blood sample may be taken, by drawing a small amount from a vein in the arm, and sent to the laboratory for tests to provide more general medical information, particularly about the possibility of inflammatory joint disease.

By injecting a local anaesthetic drug into a specific area of the spine, it can be determined whether pain arises there or not. This would be carried out by the consultant examining you or by the anaesthetist or by the consultant in the X-ray department.

Electromyography may be ordered in some hospitals if the doctor suspects damage to the nerve root. It is done to test the function of the nerves supplying muscles. With an electromyograph, the electrical activity generated by muscles can be amplified and the resulting signals heard on a loudspeaker, shown on a screen or recorded. If the nerve which supplies a muscle is damaged, inflamed or its blood supply is restricted, electrical activity may arise spontaneously in the muscle and by electromyography it may be possible to identify which nerve root is involved. To listen to a muscle, a fine needle electrode has to be inserted. It involves pin pricks, but is normally not painful. Individual muscles may protest and, if so, it helps the doctor to be told what you notice. However, any pain caused is brief and leaves no after-effects. Each time the electrode is inserted, the doctor may want you to use the muscle so that he can listen to the noise it makes. Then he will ask you to relax, so that he can listen for spontaneous activity. He may in addition do other tests to measure the speed with which nerves conduct the impulses in response to stimulation.

—special radiological investigations

In some cases, the consultant may want to have special X-rays carried out for which you will need to be admitted to hospital for a couple of days. Many surgeons will insist on some such investigation before deciding whether or not to recommend an operation.

The two main methods of getting more data from radiographs by using a contrast medium (liquid which shows up on X-rays) are myelography in which the medium fills and outlines the inside of the dural tube, and discography in which it is injected into the disc to show the extent, if any, of disruption of the nucleus.

In *myelography*, the contrast medium is injected into the dural tube inside the spinal canal. Using an image-intensifying screen, the radiologist can then see anything bulging into the canal, such as a prolapsed disc or a degenerated joint, which shows up as an indentation on the dural tube or an obliteration of part of a dural root sleeve.

The contrast medium (generally an oily one) is injected by lumbar puncture under local anaesthesia and a sample of cerebro-spinal fluid is taken for routine laboratory testing. This is done in the ward by one of the house surgeons or registrars, or the radiologist may do it when you get to the X-ray department.

For the actual investigation, you lie on a table which can be raised to the vertical so that the radiologist can observe the movement of the contrast medium in the dural tube as you are tilted up and down. The table may also tilt sideways, or the apparatus rotate in relation to the table, so that the radiologist can view the spine from different angles. He will probably take still radiographs to record the significant findings. Most of the time, however, he will be studying the picture on a television monitor which you may be able to see, too. If a large quantity of oily contrast medium has been used, it will be removed using the same type of needle to withdraw it as for injecting it.

When the myelography is finished, you will be returned to the ward, with instructions to lie quietly for up to 24 hours in order to avoid getting a severe headache.

Discography may show something which does not appear on a myelogram. It consists of an injection into the centre of discs. Generally, the three lower lumbar discs are all injected. Injecting a healthy disc is painless, but an injection into the disc which is the cause of the trouble will produce the pain. Only a small quantity of water-soluble contrast medium is used, and the patient does not have to be tipped about. In a healthy disc, the medium stays discretely in the middle but in a degenerated one it spreads out, and it may show the extent and direction of any prolapse.

Radiculography is a type of myelography which is better for showing the nerve root sleeves (radicula is the latin word for small root). Instead of an oily contrast medium, a water-soluble one is used which penetrates the root sleeves more deeply and shows more. Its main advantage, apart from clearer pictures of the nerve roots, is that it dissolves away and, unlike the oily media, leaves no traces to obscure the picture in future radiographs. The main disadvantage of some water-soluble media is that they must not be allowed to run up the spinal canal because, although quite safe around the nerve roots, they can irritate the spinal cord. Afterwards, you will be told to rest quietly for 24 hours but not to lie flat for the first six hours.

There are some other alternative radiological investigations for someone with severe symptoms or repeated attacks (these investigations are the exception rather than the rule for uncomplicated cases of back and sciatic pain). For example, the root itself can be injected outside the spinal canal—*extraspinal radiculography*. The epidural space can be injected via the gap between the bones of the sacrum and coccyx to show the space in the spinal canal surrounding the dural tube—*epidurography*. Alternatively, the medium can be injected direct into the bone of the spinous process and drains into the veins of the epidural space—*epidural venography*. Contrast medium can be injected into one of the lumbar arteries to show how rich the blood supply is locally—*lumbar arteriography*. Occasionally, *tomograms* are taken to show details in one special plane of the spine. For this, you will be asked to lie still on the table while the X-ray tube and the screen are swung in opposite directions either side of you. In *stereoradiography*, X-rays are taken to give three-dimensional effect.

Psychological aspects

Increasingly it is recognised that persistent back pain is a profoundly disturbing experience. If it goes on long enough, it may cause a genuine depression and disturb the normal pattern of behaviour, quite secondarily to the back pain. Some people seem to adapt well to their pain and build a new pattern of life around it.

For a given spinal disorder, people tend to react differently. This reflects differences in personality, and doctors are now coming to realise that it is helpful to know more about this. Some people can tolerate a lot of pain and others only a little; under stress, some of us may become anxious, hypochondriacal or depressed. Which of these characteristics will be produced when we are under stress is relevant to pain and how it affects us.

Someone with chronic and persistent pain may be given routine psychometric tests. These mostly consist of filling in a form by putting ticks in appropriate boxes in reply to lists of questions, and of tests for pain tolerance in which measurements are taken of how much (and for how long) harmless discomfort a person can tolerate.

It is because of psychological differences between people that patients with similar X-rays, similar physical states, similar diseases, react differently, not only to their condition but also to their treatment. In addition, different chemical, hormonal, vascular, nervous and other responses may occur from apparently identical doses of simple drugs so that a series of initially similar situations may lead to a variety of final results.

It is therefore important that the person treating a patient should do his or her best to treat the whole patient. In order to achieve this, there needs to be a degree of rapport and mutual cooperation between the patient and the doctor—and this also applies to physiotherapists, occupational therapists, osteopaths, and everyone else concerned. In some cases, minor physical complaints may be exaggerated in the patient's mind either consciously or unconsciously until they produce a quite disproportionate disability and then the person may need as much treatment to the mind as to the body.

Innumerable treatments for back pain have been tried over the centuries, ranging from having your back walked upon by the seventh son of a seventh son, to the application of brown paper and a smoothing iron.

Because the actual site and cause of the pain are not easy to identify, treatments have been largely empirical and therefore vary enormously. There is no scientific body of knowledge which allows the doctor to state with certainty that a particular treatment will cure the pain. Nor is there enough information to predict the treatment which will give best results. Most acute episodes of back pain get better whatever treatment is given (or even if none is given). This is probably because the pain is usually due to mild injury and, like mild injury anywhere, gets better naturally with rest.

Basically, the treatment which is currently offered by doctors starts with conservative, non-surgical, methods and then, if necessary, goes on to surgical treatment. Fashions come and go far more easily when too little is known about diagnosis and treatment, but advances are beginning to be made as a result of research, and when diagnosis becomes more accurate, treatment can be more logically designed.

Conservative treatment
The simplest way of coping with back pain is to avoid the postures and movements which cause the pain. This treatment is what the general practitioner commonly advises, in the first instance. It is based on the premise that where there is no serious disease, the inflammatory process will settle if aggravating factors

are removed. This may mean not going to work, leaving some chores undone and, if necessary, staying in bed.

The doctor may prescribe pills: painkillers, relaxants, anti-inflammatory drugs, sleeping pills.

The commonest painkillers in use are salicylates in various forms (mainly acetyl salicylic acid: aspirin), paracetamol and dextropropoxyphene; also mixtures of these and other drugs such as codeine phosphate. For more intractable pain, pentazocine, dihydrocodeine tartrate, or pethidine may be ordered; these need a doctor's prescription.

(These names are the names of the drugs themselves, not the brand names that drug manufacturers use for individual drugs and the mixtures that they combine in a single pill. But the contents should be on the label.)

Relaxants are another line of approach. They are intended to relax the back muscles which tend to be held unnecessarily tense, if not in spasm, when there is pain, so making the pain worse. Amongst relaxant drugs that may be prescribed are diazepam, meprobamate and methocarbamol.

Drugs are also used to reduce inflammation. Chief and most useful of all anti-inflammatory drugs is acetyl salicylic acid. Others in regular use are aloxiprin, benorylate, flufenamic acid, ibuprofen, indomethacin, mefenamic acid, oxyphenbutazone, phenylbutazone—and many others.

Sleeping pills are often prescribed for people whose back pain prevents sleep, and it can be useful to combine a painkiller with a sleeping pill.

Few medicines have only the single effect of relieving your symptoms. What you have to remember about any pill or combination of pills prescribed for you is that it or they may have side effects. Often, the side effect does not matter—for instance, a dry mouth. Many of these drugs tend to constipate, which will not matter if it is only for a few days; others may upset the stomach or make you dizzy or fuddled, and that could be worse than the backache. Although there is a standard dose for all these pills, some people require either more or less than the usual. What you need is just enough to produce the desired effect. If it does not produce the desired effect or if the unpleasantness (or danger) of the side effect is greater than the benefit, then stop taking the drug. You should report what has happened to the doctor and ask if he can find an alternative for you.

corsets and other supports

Abdominal and spinal supports of many different types are supplied through the national health service. They may be made of fabric, like corsets, or of other materials. The general practitioner cannot prescribe these but has to send you to the hospital for the consultant to prescribe. A small charge is made for fabric supports except for anyone who can claim exemption. (Details of exemptions can be obtained at the hospital.) No charge is made for spinal supports or braces made from materials other than fabric—for example, leather, steel, plastic, plaster-of-paris.

For an acute attack, you may be supplied with an 'instant' corset—one which comes in a few standard sizes and is seldom deeper than 12 inches. It has either buckles or velcro fastening so that it can be pulled tight round the hip bones and lumbar region. Instant means that it is handed to you in the outpatient department, without your having to wait to have one made to measure.

For more persistent pain or perhaps after an operation, you may be prescribed a tailored fabric corset or other lumbar support. General hospitals arrange for corsets to be made by surgical appliance manufacturers, but some orthopaedic hospitals have their own appliance department, and some lumbar supports and cervical collars may be made in the occupational therapy or physiotherapy department. Corsets are made to measure for the individual, and the consultant is responsible for ensuring that each completed appliance conforms to the prescription and is satisfactory in manufacture, fit and function when fitted on the patient. It takes a few weeks for a corset to be fitted and ready to wear.

The design of corsets varies considerably. Most of them are stiffened at the back: with steel reeds, for instance, which are bent to suit your contours. Women's corsets can be fitted well up to the rib cage. They are often made with laces to allow for minor changes in girth and so ensure that the corset can always be fastened tightly. For men, corsets are usually made less long, with stronger belt support round the hip bones.

As far as is known, lumbar supports are successful because they adjust the patient's method of lifting, sparing the painful area. They act as a training device to encourage correct lifting and bending—for example, they should interfere with bending at the waist, and make the patient bend at the knees. Also, a firm support round the lower back and abdomen increases intra-abdominal pressure and this increase in pressure protects the spine in all lifting actions and exertions involving the trunk.

A full-length tailored corset is likely to be prescribed when forward movement of the spine needs to be limited, where there is persistent pain or when the abdominal muscles are very weak. Such a corset does not improve poor muscular support but supplements it. Its stiffness limits backward movement, but it will only limit forward movement if it is tight enough round the chest, abdomen and hip to hold you against the steels. The fabric itself may limit sideways movements and rotation, but this depends on how high the corset comes. Some people wear one for years, and would feel lost without it.

A corset does not necessarily have to be worn all the time. You should ask for specific instructions about when and for how long you should wear yours. The support may well be taken off at night or worn only when the back is most likely to be troublesome. You may be able to progress from full-time to part-time wearing of any support. It is inadvisable to wear it for longer than your doctor intends. This is because muscles may become weak, or even weaker, if their function of supporting the spine is taken over by the corset.

Usually patients are given only one support or corset at a time. Many fabric supports can be washed;

some corsets need dry cleaning, but it is sometimes difficult to get cleaners to accept them. You should ask about this problem when the corset is being fitted. If you have been prescribed a corset or lumbar support which you must continue to wear constantly, you should ask the hospital for a spare one. Do not try to manage with only one. The NHS supplies appliances in duplicate when the provision of two is necessary on medical or hygienic grounds. So, if you need a second corset, you do not have to get one made up privately. In the course of time, you may also need a spare to wear if one has gone back to the hospital for repairs.

The hospital will repair your corset whenever this is needed, although you may find it quicker to do minor repairs to straps and to the pockets which hold the steels yourself. There is no definite period after which you are entitled to another new corset. Much depends on the circumstances and disability of the wearer. Each hospital interprets the regulations in its own way. For example, one hospital may decide that when the cost of a repair exceeds 60 per cent of the cost of a new appliance, repair is uneconomical and a new appliance can be ordered. Others may expect appliances to last for two years, and take some persuading to prescribe a new appliance in under that time.

Stronger and more rigid spinal supports are also available. This might be a plaster-of-paris (p.o.p.) jacket or a spinal brace made like a steel cage. Plaster-of-paris would be used on a short-term basis, a spinal brace where a more supportive appliance is

needed for a longer period. Plaster-of-paris does not
give as readily as fabric so it cannot be fitted as low
as a fabric corset, otherwise it would cut into the
thighs when sitting down. Alternatively, a moulded
plastic jacket may be supplied, which is considerably
lighter and quicker to fit (but warm to wear).

For a plaster-of-paris jacket the plaster is put on
wet, then dries into shape. It takes about 24 hours to
harden properly. The jacket is not easily damaged,
except by water. It has to be worn for anything from
four weeks to up to three months.

Physiotherapy
Some hospitals allow general practitioners to send
patients direct to the hospital physiotherapy department; in most, the patient has to go via the outpatient
clinic. The doctor referring a patient for physiotherapy sends with the patient the necessary particu-
lars of the person and the condition, with suggestions
and requests for treatment.

The recognised training for a physiotherapist in
this country is a three-year course at one of the
schools of physiotherapy attached to hospitals. A
student who passes the examinations qualifies for
membership of the Chartered Society of Physiotherapy and for state registration. State registered and
chartered physiotherapists are bound by their professional code of conduct to treat only patients
referred to them by a doctor. Only state-registered
physiotherapists can work within the national health
service. Physiotherapists work in hospitals, in local
authority clinics, in special schools, in industry and

sports, and also in private practice. It is not a closed profession (anyone can set up in practice as a physiotherapist) but only those who have passed the examinations of the Chartered Society of Physiotherapy can put MCSP after their name, and those who are state-registered SRP.

Physiotherapy uses physical methods to restore the function of the body and rehabilitate the patient so that he or she may return to as active and independent a life as possible.

As far as back trouble is concerned, the main methods of physical treatment are therapeutic movement or exercises, traction, massage and manipulative procedures. There are various forms of heat treatment, such as radiant heat—the sort you get from sitting in front of a fire or radiator—or short wave diathermy in one form or another, which warms the tissues in depth. Ultrasonic therapy, a form of high frequency sound energy, may be used to relieve stiffness deep in the tissues. Alternatively, ice packs may be used, particularly if there is some osteoarthrosis in your spine.

More than one method of treatment may be tried at any one time; each patient's condition and progress is reassessed regularly, and the treatment altered accordingly. For example, a patient with very acute back pain may initially be given heat treatment and an instant support to wear. This may be followed after a couple of days by traction or gentle mobilisation, and possibly later by a vigorous manipulation, and the treatment completed by a regime of exercises and instruction on how to lift safely. What a patient does when not having treatment plays an important role in recovery, therefore ask the physiotherapist what you should do between treatments.

—exercises

Exercises prescribed for you will be designed to mobilise and to strengthen—there is no point in having a range of movement without adequate muscular control. Back and abdominal muscles may become weak if they are not used for any length of time or because of pain. Muscle weakness can itself be a source of pain when what normally is a gentle physical activity leads to strain or injury. Lying in bed for a week would make you unfit to resume any heavy work immediately; four weeks' inactivity would have an even more weakening effect, possibly requiring a week's exercises to regain strength.

The physiotherapist may give any of a number of different exercises, depending on the patient's condition and how fit he needs to be to return to normal life. What is right for one patient is not necessarily correct for another, but some of the more usual exercises that a patient may come across in the physiotherapy department include back extension, flexion, side bending and rotation. A muscle has to be made to work in order to increase its strength.

Back extension exercises are designed to strengthen and mobilise the spine when it is extended. Flexion strengthens the abdominal muscles; sideways bending and twisting helps to mobilise the spine. To do this, the physiotherapist may provide manual or other resistance to particular movements. In addition, spinal exercises are sometimes given in a swimming pool.

There is also a system of exercises which, besides mobilising and strengthening, improves neuro-muscular coordination; physiotherapists call it proprioceptive neuro-muscular facilitation (PNF).

In some physiotherapy departments, exercises are carried out in classes. Provided that you are not too bothered by the want of privacy, this has a useful competitive effect, even though individual supervision may be diluted. One of the disadvantages of a general physiotherapy class is that patients of mixed ages and physical ability may be expected to do roughly the same type of exercise. Many patients may well overdo things in their endeavour to keep up with the class. Exercises should be tailored according to the age and the needs of the individual and should not cause pain. If an exercise causes pain, it may be aggravating the condition. Do not, therefore, hesitate to point out to the physiotherapist when an exercise is painful so that she can adjust the exercises accordingly.

If you have been instructed in how to perform the exercises and are trusted to do them at home, make sure that you do do them.

postural therapy
Postural stress is a common cause of back pain but if it is dictated by existing conditions at work or at home, treatment as such may not help much. Many of us, however, acquire minor postural deformities which lead to avoidable backache and which can themselves be treated: for example, the tendency to a

rounded back, head poked forward and shoulders tensed up. If this is due to muscular weakness and stiffness, exercises should help. But often it is just a matter of habit. Old habits have therefore to be shed and new ones learned, and postural therapy can help.

There is one method called the Alexander therapeutic technique. The late F. Matthias Alexander was a specialist in healing by means of postural re-education. He treated a wide variety of people for many different kinds of symptoms including back pain. The 'Alexander principle' is based on teaching patients to relax their muscles, particularly those in the neck and shoulders, and in encouraging them to make a habit of using less stressful postures and better balanced movements. This takes time and requires detailed individual instruction at first for which a series of lessons will be needed for which you would have to pay privately. There are specialist teachers who have undergone a three-year training course under the auspices of the Society of Teachers of the Alexander Technique and a number of doctors are interested in the technique.

traction
By applying a pulling force to the spine, back pain or sciatic pain can sometimes be relieved. It is not known why it works when it does; possibly by reducing tension or spasm in the back and hip muscles. Some doctors have claimed that it reduces the bulge of a disc protrusion, but the evidence is unconfirmed. Even if prolapsed disc material could be reduced in this way, it would certainly not stay reduced. For

many people, traction is a good form of treatment. However, if it is not helping, there is no point in persisting with it.

While one end of the spine is held, traction is applied by someone else pulling on it manually or by using an apparatus. However the tractive force is applied, the patient needs to be comfortable, otherwise the muscles of the back and trunk will fail to relax and so will prevent the pull from reaching the spine itself.

Traction can also be given on a special traction table. Corset-like harnesses are fixed round your pelvis and your chest and the two pulled apart. This is done either by a ratchet device which increases the pull to between 40 and 100 lb and is left like that for about ten to thirty minutes; or intermittently, the traction being applied by an electric motor every five to ten seconds. The strength of the pull, its direction and duration will be decided by the physiotherapist, and depends on how big you are, how restricted your movements are and on how bad and where the pain is. If the traction makes the pain worse at the time, it will be stopped; if the pain is worse after traction, the treatment should be discontinued.

Someone with severe back pain may have traction given as an inpatient. Either a corset-like belt is put round the hips or adhesive plaster applied to the leg and weights (10 to 20 lb) attached and run over a pulley at the end of the bed. To prevent your being pulled off by the weights, the bed is raised at the foot. Traction will be continued for one or two weeks, or until its removal causes no return of pain.

manipulation

To manipulate is to handle. The laying-on of hands is an ancient practice, and has much more than ritual significance. A doctor cannot examine the spine or any joint without handling it, any more than he can examine muscles, tendons, ligaments or joint capsules without to some extent manipulating the soft tissues under the skin. If the handling is done with healing intent, that is manipulative treatment. In that sense, massage is manipulation. Often, however, the word manipulation is taken to mean the application of a vigorous twisting force to some part of the body. Spinal manipulation is a common form of treatment. Methods vary considerably; they each work well in suitable cases, but none of them is universally successful.

Manipulation of the soft tissues is practised with the aim of achieving muscle relaxation. Putting a joint through its range of movement is the next therapeutic stage of manipulation. The aim is to increase the active range of movement. If the joint is painful, it should be supported so that mechanical stresses—the main source of pain—are minimised. This demands skill on the part of the manipulator.

The ultimate phase of most types of manipulative therapy is 'corrective' joint manipulation. This is the application of a deliberate thrust or jerk to increase joint mobility, taking the movement a bit farther than it goes in ordinary active movement but within the normal passive range. It may be performed by an orthopaedic surgeon with the patient under anaesthesia, but more often it is done without anaesthesia.

There may be some momentary discomfort but, with skilled hands, the process should not be unduly painful.

There are several systems of manipulative technique, and each manipulator has his own favourite set of methods, which may work for you or may not. It is practically impossible to make objective comparisons of different techniques.

In what is called non-specific manipulation, the patient lies on one side on the couch and the manipulator stands in front, the patient's shoulder is pushed away and the uppermost hip thrust in the opposite direction so that the whole lumbar and thoracic spine is rotated. The patient turns on the other side and the process is repeated in the opposite direction.

Specific techniques in which the aim is to focus the application of manipulative force to a single spinal joint are taught by a number of different professional groups. Geoffrey Maitland, a physiotherapist in Australia, has designed a system of vertebral manipulation which is now standard teaching for most physiotherapists in this country. The techniques themselves are similar in many respects to osteopathic techniques, the main difference lying in the system of coding and grading the forces applied while mobilising. These are small specific oscillatory movements which range from very gentle to the sudden thrust near the limit of the range of motion.

Dr James Cyriax's methods have been taught to a number of medical practitioners and to physiotherapists. The methods are less specific in their application to spinal joints than Maitland's or the osteopathic or chiropractic techniques. Generally, greater forces are applied, and for some manoeuvres an assistant is needed to hold the patient.

Doctors can join the British Association of Manipulative Medicine which runs courses in manipulative techniques for registered medical practitioners who are interested in using manipulation as a method of treatment.

Osteopathy, chiropractic and naturopathy
A number of professional groups practise physical therapy, including manipulation. Their treatment is not normally available on the national health service. You do not need to go through your doctor to see an osteopath, chiropractor or naturopath but can consult one direct on your own responsibility. However, although he should tell you if your condition is not suitable for his treatment and ought to be seen by a doctor, it might be wise to consult your doctor beforehand to ensure that there is no medical contra indication in your case.

An osteopath or any other manipulator is not allowed to prescribe drugs listed under the Dangerous Drugs Act unless he is also a registered medical practitioner. Osteopathic and chiropractic training includes the use of X-rays, and many practitioners have their own X-ray equipment. There is a DHSS code of practice for protection against ionising radiations arising from medical use.

Like doctors in private practice, osteopaths, naturopaths and chiropractors can charge whatever fees they choose. It is wise, therefore, to ask beforehand what the charge is likely to be for your course of treatment.

—osteopaths

Osteopathic manipulation of the spine is designed to be applied specifically to a particular joint segment of the spine, focussing the application of manipulative force on the range of motion between an individual pair of vertebrae. This may be done simply by applying the force directly to the vertebra concerned. More often, however, the technique is to lock the vertebrae on either side of the joint and then, using the movement of the patient's body to provide momentum, apply a corrective thrust.

Osteopathic techniques are practised by osteopaths trained in this country or in the USA (where in most states the training is comparable with medical training), by medical practitioners and by other healers who have taught themselves. In this country, training in osteopathic methods is provided by the British School of Osteopathy, which runs four-year full-time diploma courses for people without medical qualifications wishing to train as osteopaths, and by the London College of Osteopathy whose one-year course is designed for qualified doctors who can then become licentiates of the College (LLCO). Someone who has completed one of these courses (or an american doctor of osteopathy) can become a member of the Register of Osteopaths and the letters MRO after an osteopath's name indicate membership of the Register.

There is an Osteopathic Association of Great

Britain consisting mainly of registered osteopaths, and an Osteopathic Medical Association for doctors interested in osteopathy.

Osteopathic techniques are practised in this country not only by trained osteopaths and by medical practitioners who have taken courses in osteopathy, but also by practitioners who are self-taught. The letters DO (diploma in osteopathy) on their own after someone's name may mean only a diploma obtained by post from a correspondence school, but they are also used by some graduates of the British School of Osteopathy and by those who hold an american doctoral degree in osteopathy.

—chiropractors

Chiropractors, who concentrate on the spine, use a somewhat different range of manipulative techniques to osteopaths, although there are some features common to both. Chiropractic manipulation, or adjustment of the spine, is aimed at specific joints. The leverage technique is generally applied with the patient prone, supine or sitting. The recoil techniques demand the use of a special adjustable treatment table, with the patient prone.

Few medical practitioners or physiotherapists have had chiropractic training but, as with osteopathy, many develop skills which have a chiropractic basis. A chiropractor who has taken a full-time training course at a college of chiropractic in this country or in the USA can become a member of the British Chiropractors' Association and be on its register, and may put the letters DC after his name.

—naturopaths

Naturopaths also practise manipulative techniques. A naturopath treats ailments on the basis that healing depends on the correct action of the natural curative forces within the human organism. Naturopaths discourage treatment by drugs and advocate correct diet and regulated activities as the means of maintaining good health.

The letters ND (or by some DO) after a practitioner's name indicate that he has done a four-year full-time course in naturopathy and osteopathy at the British Naturopathic and Osteopathic College, and MBNOA that he is a member of the BNO Association, open only to those who have trained at the College. The Association publishes a register of its practitioner members.

Injection therapy

In some cases, the doctor injects a local anaesthetic drug into painful areas of the spine where the pain appears to be localised. This helps to identify the site of origin of the pain. Either a longer-lasting anaesthetic drug can then be injected locally, or steroids such as hydrocortisone acetate or prednisolone. Some doctors inject a sclerosing agent.

The common method is to give an epidural injection—that is, into the spinal canal in the area between the dural tube and the walls of the canal. Usually, a quantity of dilute local anaesthetic drug is followed by a steroid to reduce inflammation round the dural tube and nerve roots. The injection is at the base of the sacrum and the drugs diffuse rapidly up the canal and to the intervertebral foramina. In some hospitals, epidural injections are given in the outpatient department, although a patient may be kept in hospital just for the day to get a few hours' rest. If the injection is done under anaesthesia, manipulative treatment may be given at the same time, and then the patient is usually kept in overnight.

disc injections

A new method of treatment called discolysis or chemonucleolysis is now being offered in this country. An enzyme—chymopapain—is injected into the nucleus of the disc. It has the effect of dissolving the more complex proteins in the nucleus and in prolapsed parts of the nucleus. Afterwards, the disc may appear to be perceptibly narrower and be stiffer. Because of this reduction in volume, the mechanical

E

effects of a prolapsed disc are reduced.

The criteria for discolysis are the same, broadly speaking, as those for an operation for removal of a disc prolapse: a history of back pain with pain down the leg diagnosed as due to a prolapsed disc involving one of the nerve roots. The method has not been subjected to a controlled clinical trial but the results are about the same for discolysis as for surgery but without the risks intrinsic to surgery.

Discolysis is done in the X-ray department, generally but not always under anaesthesia. The orthopaedic surgeon or neurosurgeon first injects some contrast medium into the disc to assess the amount of degenerative change; then, with the needle still in place, injects the chymopapain. If successful, the pain in the leg goes, sometimes dramatically. However, most patients have some backache for a week or two.

acupuncture

Acupuncture is used in China for the relief of pain. In this country it has been studied in a small group of patients with intractable pain in the leg due to severe mechanical derangements of the spine, for whom an operation or further operations were thought inexpedient, and in several the pain was eased. At present, acupuncture is available only from private practitioners. The Acupuncture Association keeps a register of trained acupuncturists. Members of the Medical Acupuncture Society are doctors trained in acupuncture. A report on acupuncture was published in *Which?* February 1972.

Surgical treatment

No guarantee is ever given beforehand by a surgeon that a spinal operation will be a success. However, the majority are successful—otherwise surgeons would not continue doing them. The surgeon should discuss the position with you fully beforehand, and give you some idea of what to expect after the operation. No operation is done without the patient's consent. A surgeon is unlikely to suggest an operation unless he is fairly sure of your full cooperation at all stages. To a large extent, the success of the operation will depend on your determination to regain strength and get back to normal.

There are three main reasons for operating: to relieve mechanical stress on the lumbar and sacral nerve roots; to stabilise one or more adjacent intervertebral joints when there is a mechanical weakness locally; and for intractable pain.

Sometimes the surgeon cannot be certain that he will only have to remove a prolapsed disc or only have to stabilise with a bone graft (spinal fusion). Very often he has to explore to find the cause of pain: this exploratory operation is called lumbar spondylotomy.

The name often—and usually incorrectly—used to describe a spinal operation is laminectomy, which just means removal of the lamina, the bony shelf in the vertebral arch. But the word is often used to refer to almost any kind of operation on the spine.

In spinal surgery to free the nerve root, removal of prolapsed disc material (discectomy) may be all that is necessary. This is usually done by making a window (fenestration) in the ligamentum flavum and if necessary nibbling away a bit of the lamina to improve surgical access. It is not a serious operation and you may be allowed up in a few days, encouraged to walk and to bend, and soon be back at work.

But sometimes it is necessary to remove from the vertebral arch or body, bony thickening and osteophytes if they are found to cause stretching, angulation, adhesion, or compression of the nerve roots. (Facetectomy means the removal of bone from the articular processes of the vertebral arch.)

If much bone has to be removed, the surgeon may decide to do a spinal fusion as well, particularly when large amounts of the vertebral arch have to be removed to free the nerve roots, or to decompress the cauda equina itself inside the dural tube. But the decision to do a spinal fusion cannot always be made in advance.

—spinal fusion

Spinal fusion is designed to stiffen a section of the spine, in order to prevent a deformity such as spondylolisthesis from increasing; to fix a section where movement is painful, such as a degenerated disc giving an abnormal pattern of movement with secondary changes in the synovial joints; or to stabilise the spine in an area weakened during surgery, as in cases where bone has had to be removed to free the nerve roots.

Most commonly, the operation consists of the laying down of a bone graft to increase the bony stability of the spine across one, two or three segments. The bone for fusion is almost invariably taken from the back of the hip bone. This leaves no deformity or weakness and provides enough healthy bone which is readily accessible during spinal surgery. Fusion can be performed by laying the bone graft at the back of the arch to each side and at the side of the synovial joints, or between the vertebral bodies after removing the whole of the disc. In some cases, in order to hold the fused joints steady while the bone graft is consolidating, the surgeon will add further stability by inserting metal screws, plates, clips or coil springs.

Until a few years ago, spinal fusion meant lying in a plaster shell for a month and in bed for up to three months before being allowed up. Nowadays, however, this is less common. Some surgeons allow patients up when they feel like it, provided there is nothing to contra-indicate this. However, a typical post-operative course following a spinal fusion is for the patient to lie flat in bed for up to three weeks, with no more than two pillows and with instructions to avoid lying curled up. When allowed out of bed, he must avoid low chairs, must not sit with legs out straight, should avoid bending. He will be given a tailored corset or a plaster-of-paris jacket to wear, and will be advised to take exercise by walking. Three months or so after the operation, the patient will probably be given exercises by the physiotherapist to start mobilising the spine and strengthen the muscles. After six months, he could be back to full activity. But many patients go on improving for well over a year. A lot depends on the patient. The back muscles may take quite a while to recover from the operation and to regain normal strength. The physiotherapist will show the way but it is the patient who has to do the work.

—rhizolysis

Rhizolysis is a comparatively new form of surgical treatment which involves a series of small incisions with a lancet through the skin over the synovial joints of the lumbar region. The aim is to cut the nerve which supplies the synovial joints. This, it is said, will relieve the back pain. It assumes that the pain arises from the joints and that the nerves are indeed cut. The difficulty is that the particular nerves cannot be seen when the cutting is attempted, and, in any event, the synovial joint is supplied from other nerves which are less accessible. So the procedure is questionable. There are some new ways of doing it, using electric methods, but none has been subjected to a controlled trial.

Occupational therapy

After surgery, or after a prolonged and disabling spell of pain, a patient may be referred to the occupational therapy department for rehabilitation. After some forms of surgery, patients need help and advice on everyday activities such as dressing and bathing—for example, it may be necessary to kneel, not sit, in the bath.

Patients are referred to occupational therapy in the same way as they are referred to physiotherapy. The two aspects of treatment are likely to overlap. Usually the physiotherapist treats the patient in the earlier stage, and the occupational therapist when the time has come to re-educate patterns of movement in order to avoid back strain in the future.

Occupational therapy is a state registered profession and occupational therapists who have completed their three-year training are entitled to put SROT after their name. MBAOT indicates membership of the British Association of Occupational Therapists.

Occupational therapy is requested in the first instance by the consultant. The actual treatment is left to the discretion of the occupational therapist. It may take the form of any activity, work or recreation chosen specifically for the individual patient to aid his recovery and resettlement, or to minimise the effects of a permanent disability and to help him to live with such a disability. Patients benefit by working at both occupational therapy and physiotherapy. Some people prefer to be in a workshop, while others respond better in a gymnasium, and their programme may be adapted accordingly.

When the time comes for considering a return to work, the occupational therapist will analyse the patient's job and prescribe tasks within the occupational therapy department which equate as far as possible with what he will need to do, whether the occupation involves heavy physical work or prolonged sitting in the same position, or working in awkward positions or lifting heavy weights. The occupational therapist will observe to see whether the patient is putting into practice what he has been taught. However good your intentions may be, it is all too easy to slip back into the habits of a lifetime when you are trying to get your work done.

In nearly all occupational therapy departments there is an area with a kitchen, a bathroom and a bedroom, where a woman who is mainly a housewife is asked to try out the correct technique for household jobs, under supervision, and then repeats each task over a period of time so that she becomes conditioned automatically to save her back.

If the house you live in is badly designed for a person with back trouble, the occupational therapist from the hospital, or one from the local authority social services department, may visit and make recommendations on adaptations that may help. The social services department may be able to provide financial help to carry them out.

Rehabilitation and convalescence
There are a number of employment rehabilitation centres throughout the country to which patients, particularly men whose work requires physical strength, can be sent, as inpatients or outpatients depending on locality. There, physiotherapy and remedial gymnastic therapy is allied to practice at the type of work to which the patient hopes to return. This can be valuable particularly for those working in industries in which no provision is made for someone requiring a temporary spell of light work.

Alternatively, there are convalescent homes to which patients can go following surgery or prolonged disability, at which physiotherapy is available. The atmosphere is gentler and there is not the same emphasis on return to hard work. The social worker at the hospital can make the arrangements at the consultant's request.

Some people have had to be told that there is no more to be offered by way of treatment for their back trouble, that they cannot be given a new spine and that they must learn to live with it. Even after a reassurance that there is no serious disease, such advice can be depressing, just as chronic pain itself is depressing. Some people's lives are restricted, often dominated, by their back. Many people can make the best of such a situation and learn to cope.

Some sufferers feel that there is always a chance that another surgeon, another doctor may have something to offer. Although a number of the acknowledged experts do see patients privately, the general pattern of private treatment for back pain is dominated by those who are exponents of a particular line of treatment and who therefore are unlikely to offer alternatives. The main advantage in seeing someone privately is that you are buying more time with the particular practitioner. Many people make regular visits to osteopaths simply to keep mobile, and there is probably no reason why they should not continue.

Most preventive measures are scientifically untested, though this does not mean that these methods may not one day be proved of value. 'Miracle' cures are mainly anecdotal; but if a man says that he has never felt his back since he took to eating sorrel in his salad, it would be silly to dissuade him.

Although a patient may have been told that all the normal conservative measures have been tried, there is always a possibility that the verdict may become outdated by new knowledge, improved diagnostic techniques and methods of treatment not previously available. For instance, there are now pain relief clinics in some areas where new methods of pain relief are being developed by specialist teams.

When treatment for back pain is only partially successful, or there is a spinal disorder for which the patient is told that nothing more can be done surgically, treatment of a psychological kind can sometimes help. Operant conditioning, which began in the USA, is a new kind of treatment for patients whose pain seems to be reinforced by events and who keep having to take painkillers. The treatment is carried out in an orthopaedic or rehabilitation ward or in a residential centre where the environment is controlled. The medical team includes a psychologist, a physiotherapist, an occupational therapist. Drug therapy is designed so that the patient never has to ask for painkillers, while physical activites are encouraged and increased under strict supervision. Whereas the patient had come to expect that the pain would be worse on certain occasions, which reinforced the pain, under the regime of operant conditioning the learning process is reversed so that activities and occasions come to be associated with freedom from pain, and gradually the need for painkillers diminishes.

the chronic sufferer
A chronic back sufferer can do much to help himself. First of all, there are almost certainly alternative ways of tackling any particular job which cause less spinal stress and are therefore less painful, and which are physically more efficient. Also, it is possible to alter or redesign your working environment with the aim

of minimising postural stress on the spine: by adjusting the height of a working surface, by changing your own posture, by choosing a different chair or desk. And there are a number of aids to back comfort, some designed for the disabled, which can be used to make life more independent. (The Disabled Living Foundation, 346 Kensington High Street, London W14 8NS can provide information on what special equipment is available and where it can be obtained.)

Chronic and persistent back pain can have a devastating effect on sexual activity, not only because of the pent-up sexual energy of the individual with pain but because of the partner's. The situation deserves understanding and sympathetic analysis on both sides. If it is simply that the active movements or the postures themselves are painful, a solution is possible. A soft and yielding mattress is not the best support for a painful back and if a pillow under the small of the back does not help, try firmer ground. Back pain brought on merely by the active movements can be solved by reversing the active role. The main point is to use your ingenuity and common sense. The solution may be less than perfect, it may not be what you are used to or you may have to try some totally unfamiliar technique, but it is probably better than continued abstinence. If the intensity of the orgasm itself is the trigger for pain, this is more difficult. Possibly it can be controlled by using gentler methods without so steep a crescendo. If not, it may help to take a painkiller about half an hour before foreplay. Some people claim to be able to achieve a slow and prolonged orgasm lasting twenty minutes or more, and such techniques may suit you. For those who find that the pain is dominant after rather than during, the problem is one which can only be solved empirically. It is not a bad idea to refer to a book on sexual technique if you have not already done so.

One of the problems of disabling back pain is having to give things up. What matters more than anything else here is your attitude of mind. Some people may relish the attention for which their symptoms call; most are made wretched by their physical dependency. The doctor's advice to a patient in an acute attack to avoid the activities and postures that hurt is fair and acceptable. But to someone who has been in pain for months, such advice seems meaningless particularly when almost anything hurts.

It is more important to identify positively the things that do not make matters worse, and to concentrate on them as a basis for improvement, however modest. Assuming you can find some activity—such as walking or swimming, or simple exercises—which does not upset your back, do it regularly, a bit more and a bit faster or farther every day. Any exercise will do to start as the basis for improvement. Only thus can you expect to become generally more physically fit. Those who are physically fit are generally able to tolerate pain better than the unfit. Their sensation of pain may be no different but it affects them less and they are better able to ignore it.

Without physical activity, the body becomes weak and unstable, and without movement it becomes stiff. The mobility of the spine and the resilience of its tissues are essential functions and without them the spine would be more readily strained and would lose its shock-absorbing capacity. Even more important are the muscles: not only those of the back but all which support the spine, including the abdominals. Without muscular support, the spine is unstable and easily injured.

Episodes of back pain are more likely when physical work has been heavy enough to give a feeling of effort or has led to unexpected stress. In particular, the unaccustomed, isolated, heavy task is a potential risk. Common sense will warn you that moving ten tons of coal is a job for someone who is both trained and in training for it. But in daily life one needs to be prepared for the occasional stress of humping something out of the boot of the car or moving the furniture for spring-cleaning and other odd jobs for which one is out of practice but which are sure to crop up once in a while. The question is how to keep reasonably fit for them.

You devote quite a bit of the day, in total, to keeping your skin and hair clean and presentable—so spare some time also to keep your back in reasonable working order. Many protest that they are active all day anyway and that this should keep them fit and that housework, shopping, gardening and everything else leave no time for getting unfit. No doubt it is possible to get through a busy day with a stiff back, poor abdominal muscles and hips with a third of the normal range of movement—but only after a fashion and with no reserves for the extra effort that may be needed when things go wrong.

For those who are prepared to do their 'daily dozen' either routinely or after the stimulus of a spell of backache, there are exercises which are easy to perform and take only a short time to do, plus some clear floor space. Some of them mobilise the spine, others strengthen the muscles, and some help to keep the hips and knees supple and strong—a prerequisite for safe methods of lifting and handling and for avoiding postural stress when working near to floor level.

Our postural habits are dictated by furniture, clothing, working conditions and transport, as well as by social custom. Seats and chairs are universal so that we do not need to get down to the floor, with the result that we cease to use our hips and spines as our ancestors did, although, genetically, there is nothing to stop us. Clothes, such as tight skirts or jeans and carefully creased trousers, positively restrict the potential range of movement and prevent one bending one's knees properly for lifting or holding the weight close to one's body. You cannot avoid the postural stress of stooping to do a job near floor level if your clothing and shoes prevent you from kneeling comfortably at a convenient height or if you are too stiff to sit cross-legged on the floor. Moreover, sinks, benches and other working heights are such that we spend much of the day leaning forwards with the spine posturally stressed. Simple, common sense application of ergonomic principles can relieve some postural stress. And making better use of the body's strength and range of motion will reduce much of the physical stress of modern life.

There are few advantages in being overweight. The person who is 20 pounds overweight has more weight to throw about when using the kinetic energy of the body and has perhaps only to lean on something to get it moving. But he has that much extra to carry around, a faster rate of wear and tear of weight-bearing joints, and limitation of mobility—all major disadvantages. Anyone who complains of persistent back pain but does nothing to shed excess weight will get little sympathy from the average orthopaedic surgeon—not even from a fat one.

Exercise

Two activities which create good exercise for the back are walking and swimming. Both demand spinal movement without major stress and both add to general physical fitness. Walk tall and stride evenly, whether promenading, hurrying to work or hiking; and leave the stooping, waddling plod behind. Look in a mirror or shop window when you get the chance to check that you do not walk in a crouching shuffle. Sensible shoes add to your stability; beware of fashion shoes which wobble and limit your stride. If anything heavy has to be carried, a shoulder bag or rucksack is better than a hand-held case. The extra stability or sense of rhythm provided by a walking stick or umbrella can be a help. Lifts and elevators are not really needed just for a floor or two—walk up.

Whatever is done by way of exercise wants to be a matter of routine. Cycling (but not with low handlebars —racing cyclists get backache), badminton, table and lawn tennis are all things which can be enjoyed regularly at least until you are middle-elderly, probably for longer.

—after an attack
Following a spell of back trouble, exercise of some kind is essential if weakness and stiffness are to be avoided. Simple pain-free movements of the lower limbs to be done for a few minutes every hour or so should, subject to medical approval, be begun at an early stage; the sooner the better to shorten the period of recovery. They assist the circulation and reduce the discomfort on starting to get up.

Before you can claim to be fully recovered from an attack of back pain, and provided there is nothing otherwise wrong with you, you should be able to get your knees up to your chest while sitting or lying and, while sitting, you should be able to get your shoulders down between your knees; you ought to be able to sit on the floor, for short periods anyway, with your legs out straight; you should be able to sit up from a supine position without using your arms, and should be able to squat down and rise up again with a straight back.

At some stage, you can begin taking exercise as well as doing exercises. Provided it does not cause pain and there is no medical objection, start going for walks (or swimming)—short distances to begin with, slowly increasing. Walking is particularly important after a spell of back trouble, especially if you found yourself limping a little during the attack. If you can manage to walk properly for only a short distance at a time, do it more often.

exercises

The following are exercises which will help to restore spinal mobility and to strengthen the muscles which control the movements and postures of the spine. Begin gently and do not struggle to do any that hurt; the easier ones are at the beginning of each section. For a start, the rule is to do the exercises for only a little while but fairly often. In this way, the muscles have a chance to build up gradually without becoming tired. And each time look for a little improvement in mobility and strength.

Use your common sense during these exercises and ask your doctor if you are in doubt.

The best place is on the floor. You will need a space at least six feet square, more for long-legged people. That may mean moving the furniture, for which you may need to get help. Bare boards would be too hard and if the carpet is thin, put down a couple of blankets or an old bed quilt. Also, have a chair to hold on to for some of the exercises. Do them out on the lawn if the weather is good. Do not wear anything which restricts movement.

EXERCISES

Start flat on your back with your legs wide and your arms stretched over your head, and, with a few deep breaths, relax for a minute or so. And return to this relaxing posture for a while between exercises. Make sure you do some each time from the exercises on your back (supine), lying face down (prone), on your side (right and left), standing and sitting. There are additional exercises you can do kneeling, and some hanging from a beam or doorpost. Start always with the easiest, some from each section. Then, when you are able to, progress with the less easy ones— each time performing them fractionally longer or farther.

leg—the part of the lower limb between knee and ankle

thigh—the part of the lower limb between knee and hip

Supine

a) Bend one knee up until it is just past the vertical and feels balanced; do small rhythmic up and down movements, gradually getting nearer your chest—repeat other side
(*mobilises hips and spine*)

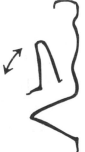

b) Bend one knee up with the foot flat on the floor about 12 inches from the side of the other knee;

Standing

Stand erect with your back straight and if necessary put your hands on a chair to steady yourself

a) Bend your knees and go up and down as far as you can while keeping your back straight—do not go too far too soon
(*strengthens knee muscles*)

b) Bend each knee up alternately, bringing them gradually nearer your chest
(*mobilises hips and spine*)

c) Bend your head down with your hands on the front of your thighs and gently slide your hands

Prone

If your back is painful, put a pillow under your belly

a) Bend your knees until the legs are vertical; gently drop your heels rhythmically up and down towards your buttocks
(*mobilises spine*)

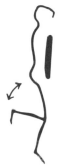

b) Bend one knee up until the leg is vertical; gently and rhythmically drop it

supine

swing the knee gently from side to side dropping it as far as it will comfortably go—repeat other side (*mobilises hips*)

c) Bend both knees up keeping feet flat on the floor; rhythmically raise and lower the small of your back, keeping buttocks and

standing

down and up, keeping your back flexed as though you were rolling and unrolling down and up. Progress steadily until you can slide your hands all the way down to your feet keeping the knees straight.

Ask your doctor if you may do this exercise in case it is inadvisable for you.

(*strengthens back muscles, mobilises hips and spine*)

d) Raise one thigh until it is horizontal and keep it so while bending and straightening the knee—repeat other side

(*strengthens knee muscles, mobilises spine*)

prone

from side to side—repeat other side (*mobilises hips*)

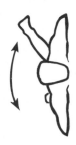

c) Bend your knees until the legs are vertical; lift thighs alternately up and down, gradually increasing the distance and number of times

(*mobilises hips and spine,*

shoulders on the floor so that your spine is alternately arched and flattened against the floor (*mobilises spine*)

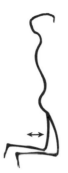

d) Bend both knees up keeping feet flat on the floor; gently raise buttocks from the floor a few times, increasing the distance you

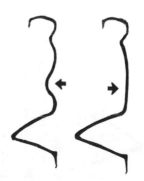

e) Alternate side bending: slide your hands up and down your thighs (*mobilises spine*)

f) With a chair for support. swing one leg with the knee straight, first backwards and forwards and then out sideways—repeat other side (*mobilises hips and spine*)

g) Stand with your feet well apart; turn body and feet to one side and gently lunge down and forward on the bent knee, keeping the other straight behind you, then up again—repeat alternate sides (*mobilises hips and spine, strengthens knee and hip muscles*)

strengthens back and hip muscles)

d) Same as (b) with legs together (*mobilises spine*)

e) Raise each leg alternately with the knee straight, slowly increasing the height (*strengthens back and hip muscles*)

f) With arms at your side and someone to hold your

supine

can lift your buttocks and the number of times (*strengthens back and hip muscles*)

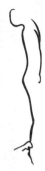

e) Same as (a) with both knees at the same time (*mobilises spine and hips*)

f) Same as (b) with both knees together (*mobilises spine and hips*)

g) Bend both knees up keeping feet flat on the floor (either with someone to hold them or with the feet

Side-lying

Each exercise to be done on each side; lie with a pillow under your head

a) Bend your uppermost knee and move it to and from your chest; then try with both knees together (*mobilises spine and hips*)

b) With the knee straight, raise leg up and down, slowly increasing the distance (*strengthens hip and trunk muscles, mobilises spine and hip*)

prone

feet, gently raise head and shoulders, progressively increasing the height lifted (*strengthens back and hip muscles*)

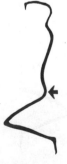

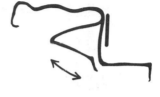

under a mattress to act as counterweight; stretch your hands forward, lift your head and shoulders to curl up as far as you can—with progress and gentle repetition you should be able to sit up
(*strengthens abdominal muscles*)

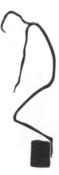

h) Same as (d) but with heels gradually farther from buttocks
(*strengthens back and hip muscles*)

Kneeling

If you have not knelt for a while, be careful not to hurt your knees

a) Sit on the floor with your knees under you and soles under your buttocks; sit tall and turn gently side to side with arms out; intersperse with deep breathing exercises, raising your arms up at each inhalation and down at each exhalation
(*mobilises spine*)

b) Kneel on all fours and, striding out quadrupedally, do a cat walk round a figure-of-eight circuit
(*mobilises spine*)

Sitting

Sit upright on a firm chair without arms, with your feet flat on the floor and your hips and knees at right angles

a) Keeping your knees bent, raise them alternately up towards your chest
(*mobilises spine and hips*)

supine

i) Bend one knee until the thigh is vertical; first, rhythmically straighten the knee with the thigh kept vertical; then putting your arms out sideways to steady yourself, swing the knee gently from side to side until it drops all the way—repeat other side

(*strengthens knee muscles and mobilises spine and hips*)

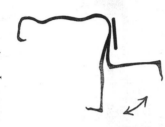

Hanging

If there is a convenient place for you to hang safely by your hands from a beam, a doorpost or the side of a staircase, you may find this relieves backache. (Some sports shops sell metal rods which can be fixed in a doorway to serve as a beam.) It does not matter if your feet are not off the floor—just put them well forward with your knees straight and relax enough for your hands to take the weight. While hanging, alternately relax with deep breathing and do some gentle knee bends to the chest.

sitting

b) Alternately straighten each knee

(*strengthens knee muscles, mobilises spine*)

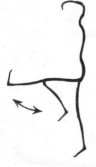

c) Set your knees well apart with your hand on each for support; then bend your

j) Same as (c) but flattening and arching the spine with legs out straight; then try pulling your heels along the floor, while keeping your spine flattened (this is not as easy as it sounds)
(*mobilises spine, strengthens hip and abdominal muscles*)

trunk up and down, progressing until you can get your shoulders down between your knees, keeping your head up
(*mobilises spine and hips*)

the end

INDEX

Coping with disablement
gives advice and information for someone disabled by increasing age or an accident or illness to help them lead as independent a life as possible about the house and outside. Many aids and techniques for dressing and carrying out everyday tasks are described, and sources of help—local authority, the health service, voluntary bodies—given.

Having an operation
describes the procedure on admission to hospital: ward routine, hospital personnel, preparation for the operation, anaesthesia, post-operative treatment, convalescence. Basic information is given about some common operations.

other Consumer Publications include:

Living through middle age
Treatment and care in mental illness
Health for old age
Care of the feet
Central heating
Getting a divorce
What to do when someone dies
Wills and probate
The legal side of buying a house
Extending your house
Pregnancy month by month
The newborn baby
Eyes right
Caring for teeth
Claiming on home, car and holiday insurance
Owning a car
Infertility
How to adopt
Arrangements for old age
Electricity supply and safety
How to sue in the county court

Consumer Publications are available from Consumers' Association, Caxton Hill, Hertford SG13 7LZ and from booksellers.